PRAISE FOR *A TINY WHITE LIGHT* . . .

"With unflinching vividness, Bass translates the logic of madness, the distortions of perception, and the sensory overload of a fractured mind not just as an experience, but as a surreal world with its own internal consistency."

—Rosie McMahan, EdM, author of *Fortunate Daughter: A Memoir of Reconciliation*

"Truly the most authentic, disturbing and riveting description of psychosis I've ever read, barring perhaps Jack Kerouac's depiction of alcoholic psychosis in his memoir *Big Sur.*"

—Dori Ostermiller, author of *Outside the Ordinary World*

"Burdened by a life marked by trauma, neglect, and solitude, Bass begins to experience a psychotic episode during psychotherapy. This book shows how what she calls "craziness" is a strategy for survival in the face of deep hurt—and a catalyst for confronting life's challenges in a new way."

—Stijn Vanheule, professor of clinical psychology at Ghent University, and author of *Why Psychosis Is Not So Crazy*

"Spanning time, place, and people, *A Tiny White Light* provides a compelling portrait of mental illness and the long, winding road of recovery."

—Maria Galano, PhD, assistant professor of clinical psychology at UMass Amherst

A TINY WHITE LIGHT

a memoir of a mind in crisis

A TINY WHITE LIGHT

Linda Bass

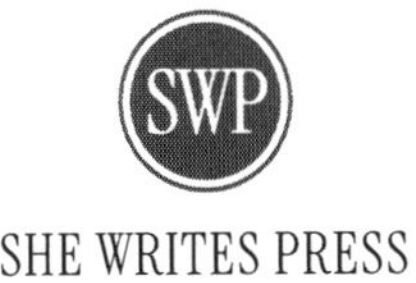

SHE WRITES PRESS

Published in 2026 by
She Writes Press, an imprint of The Stable Book Group

32 Court Street, Suite 2109
Brooklyn, NY 11201
https://shewritespress.com
Library of Congress Control Number: 2025916866
Print ISBN: 979-8-89636-044-5
eISBN: 979-8-89636-045-2

Interior Designer: Tabitha Lahr
Cover Art: Linda Bass

Printed in the United States of America

Names and identifying characteristics have been changed to protect the privacy of certain individuals.

With Love,
For Marcia
and
For Brad

AUTHOR'S NOTE

In writing this memoir, my intention was to capture the truth of my experience over forty years ago, using my journals and an early draft of this book to supplement my memories. Nevertheless, the result is a mix of my subjective truth, memories that, as we know, can evolve over time, and a bit of creative nonfiction where I paraphrased or recreated dialogue. Names of characters and identifying characteristics have been changed, as have some place names. The result is a book that reflects my version of events alone, with any inaccuracies attributable only to me.

CONTENTS

PROLOGUE:

FAMILY PORTRAIT, 1982

October 1982, a warm fall day. I sit at the long dining hall table, wearing a hospital gown, white with tiny blue flowers, and blue foam slippers, and am holding a large white sheet of construction paper and a yellow pencil, sharpened, number 2. I squint in concentration, the paper quivering in my hands, and hear the tester say, ". . . a picture of your family with each member doing something." Despite my now heavily drugged mind, I understand she will be looking for hints of family pathology, and I oddly think, *Oh, fun!* But I frown in confusion because what exactly *is* my family? I don't want to be wrong, so decide to include everybody, my family of origin and my contemporary family, figuring the right answer will be in there somewhere.

Without even thinking, I have already planned three rooms. I carefully draw the lines in perspective, splayed out to the side edges of the paper, like open legs. I pencil a door on the left wall to signify a small room, designed for a peripheral character. The right room is trickier because it must be open to view, yet separate from the central room. I make the central room an *L*, my initial, and smile, *inappropriately* the tester might be thinking, so I make my face blank again as I fashion a door for the right room so the observer may be privy to its contents: a bed, a chair.

Three enclosed rooms, with doors to each other, but no way out. One must not lose sight of the world out there—outside my head, so to speak. I draw a large central picture window on the back wall of the middle room, an eye looking out. A smaller window behind the chair in the bedroom, two eyes. There is no door out, or maybe the exit is the entire front of the picture, with its diverging lines—the only way out a flood inside my head, a widening gush into the nether regions of myself.

I replace my pencil with a cigarette. I do not want to contemplate these rooms, so I ruminate about smoke. A marching band of cigarettes walks down the hall toward me—everyone here smokes. *Fighting fire with fire*, I think. Is that one of those proverbs?

I'm more than a little worried that my leaving the hospital depends on figuring out proverbs. When my therapist, Sam, visits, he asks me to explain the meaning of "A rolling stone gathers no moss." But is it desirable for stones to be covered with moss or not? The beauty of moss—should I say that if one just rolls through life, always on the move, one is deprived of the beauty derived from sitting still and letting lovely things come to you? But maybe he wants me to think of moss as a kind of fungus, so I picture green furry moss lining my skull. Then I should say that an active life precludes some sort of decay, but I hate that notion, the idea that one should be like a stone, unthinking, unfeeling, busy, busy, going, going, gone. And then what is worth saying about one's life? The difference between being and doing, it seems to me. A value judgment.

I snuff out my cigarette. The tester is watching me, so I say, "Just taking a break." To think about moss on stones.

The picture is supposed to be of *doing*—I have been instructed to draw each family member involved in a characteristic activity. At home, in that place where I live with my husband and two children, I have an overstuffed chair that I think of as *my* chair. Antique, blue silk brocade, sprouting tufts of white cotton and some stiff brown straw-like substance that might be horsehair, although I hope not. I often sit and read in my chair—it encloses me like a cocoon. Sometimes while sitting in it, I feel hugged.

I pencil in the chair to the left of the picture window and draw my father, Dan Bailey, sitting in it. He is barrel-chested, bears an *X* on his cheek (clawed by "those damn turkeys"), and is bespectacled, looking down, silently absorbed in a book. Reading is our connection other than silence. I send him books, and in this way, we hold hands, walking into other worlds. He knows the landscapes, the people, in my head, and they live in his too. I think of us as very much alike, though I can't be sure—we rarely talk. I only imagine him, a benevolent silence.

The addendum to my father, my stepmother, is next. The peripheral character. She stands inside the door in the left room, primping her hair, holding a mirror. I pause with my pencil. Too blatant an accusation of superficiality? But all I can think of is Helma's pillow, U-shaped so her neck can rest in the valley of it and her hair remain untouched, a curlicued sculpture in white and hair spray. Helma is hard to draw, because her hair fades into the powdered white of her skin, no contrast. Jessie calls her *the white grandma*. It's too bad I can't add a soundtrack to this picture, because for my stepmother I would add a *tsk*ing noise that she forms by sucking air through her two widely spaced front teeth.

My mother is a primper too, at some of the most inauspicious times, like at my brother's funeral. Tears streaking down her face but her hand on her hair, a curved bony hand with extremely long pink fingernails. I draw her next, lying in bed in the room on the right. She is curly-headed and crying, looking straight at the observer or, more likely, at me, because I was a "mean and selfish child" who made her cry. I was also an "ideal child" who made my mother proud. Maybe I just *made* my mother up, if I was that powerful. This room has the feeling of Sunday to it. Of empty streets, no cars, Family Day. Obligatory togetherness, manufactured fun, collecting memories for evidence that something happened, passing time, losing time, a vacuum, emptiness imploding into emptiness. If this weren't a study in black and white, I'd add a wash of purple, the color of my mother's Evening in Paris perfume bottle. A touch of sadness, of lost things.

I draw my stepfather on the far side of the bedroom, sitting on a hard, spindly chair that looks as if it were picked to its bare wooden bones. He holds a rifle in one hand and a beer glass in the other. He's a hunter, shoots deer. This is *the* gun, the one my brother chose, though it's anyone's guess who should hold it in this picture. If this were a video, I'd probably have that gun tossed back and forth among most of the characters, a hot potato.

Anyway, my stepfather sits there, as if guarding my mother or holding her prisoner or maybe guarding himself—he probably doesn't know which because he is also drinking and confused. He partially blocks the eye of that room, like a lazy lid, a position that mistakenly inflates his significance, so I erase and move him to the right of the window, this time tipping his chair against the wall, the flavor of a lion tamer with the wooden legs poking into the air of the room.

In the living room, with my father, my younger sister Mandy stands at an ironing board, absorbed in her plans to go out with friends that night. As the youngest, favored, and "normal" child, she escaped much, but not all, of the kitchen-table drama.

Next I draw my children, standing front and center, closest to my heart as I lean over to draw. Jessie, four, tugs at Brandon, two, demanding his involvement in her game, while he sucks his thumb and fingers the velvety cotton of his blankie, happy enough in his self-comfort, resisting her. Brother-sister squabbling, but they touch each other, and I am glad of this. I want them to escape a pattern, to be okay.

In the picture window, I draw a road with a central broken line, like a piece of spaghetti chopped up, and a cloud, fluffy. It is simpler out there, the feel of Monday. On a motorcycle, hidden in his helmet and leathers, an armor of sorts, is my husband, leaning close to the bike, one with it. Singlemindedly pursuing nothing he sees on the empty road, but engaged in his pursuit. Rather like that rolling stone.

On the cloud, my brother lies casually on his side, legs drawn up, head resting on his hand, elbow out. A puzzle put back together, a successfully reassembled Humpty Dumpty. He is smiling, amused, above and beyond it all, maybe even laughing, just as I imagined him at his funeral, sitting atop his coffin, laughing in ridicule at the tears, at the show.

I draw myself last, sitting at my old oak desk, writing or drawing, facing the right living room wall. I cannot see my father behind me, but I know he is there, silently reading, visiting our common lands, and there is a whisper of turning pages. I hear the hiss of the steam iron as my sister daydreams. From the corners of my eyes, I see the children to my right, and to my left I can make out my brother lying one way, facing east, and my husband, the other, riding west. On the wall in front of me, blocking out my mother's face, is some artwork, pictures I will draw. I sketch in my cigarettes and an ashtray, just in case, *fire with fire*, my smoke another layer of derma, and my picture is done.

I hand my drawing to the tester but then grab it back. I have forgotten my lifeline, my connection to the real world, the umbilical cord that feeds me: my radio. I draw a caricature of a radio, just a square (the worst drawing in the picture), and I mar the portrait by printing "RADIO" across it. The requisite flaw, like my belief in those love songs. The radio plays in one corner of the desk, drowns out the quiet sobs, the pleading of the children, the distant motorcycle roar, the laughter, and the turning pages. The music surrounds me, walls of notes like skin around a private room.

I return the portrait.

The tester now questions me. “Who is who?”

I watch her print their names right over their bodies. They become cartoons like the radio. I sigh.

She asks, “What are you doing at the desk?”

“Orchestrating the lives in the picture, putting them together, composing my own kind of music, creating it note by note.”

PART I:

THE LOS ANGELES YEARS, 1967–1971

CHAPTER 1:

OUT OF THE POT, INTO THE FIRE, 1967

California. If only we'd never gone. It was where you might go to follow your dreams or to escape into anonymity, a place to shine or to misbehave without prying eyes, where it was all too easy to lose track of who you were, if you even knew in the first place, and become lost.

Our family, the Baileys, lived in a seven-room house on the edge of Houston, Wisconsin, a town of only 401 people. Sometimes our mail would end up in its big sister city in Texas. I imagined that at one time the country had been folded in two and then suddenly ripped apart, leaving just a torn remnant of Houston in Wisconsin and the majority in Texas.

Houston was a tiny country town where my friends and I could run free—swimming in the pond along with the snappers, skating on it in winter, fishing with cane poles, sleeping in someone's tree house, bicycling into the country, picking berries. But it was also stifling—the gossip, the rivalries, the provincialism, and the *uneventfulness* of it all, except for the mandatory church and school activities and all the associated expectations for good behavior and moral fiber. I, for one, couldn't wait to leave. And then my mother unintentionally made that happen.

After discovering my mother's affair with a married guy named Peter, my father still wanted to make their marriage work, and he agreed to selling his share of the turkey farm, along with our house and most of our possessions, and moving to California so my mother could be near her mother and sisters, if only she would be willing to try. She agreed.

In June 1967, our family of five, including thirteen-year-old Mandy, eighteen-year-old Brian, and nineteen-year-old me, moved to Granada Hills in the San Fernando Valley in Los Angeles.

Within weeks of our move, Peter told my mother he'd left his wife and was planning to follow her to LA. Our parents decided to divorce, after asking Brian and me what we thought, as if asking our permission or at least pretending to. I said I thought it might be a good thing—maybe they'd both be happier—while Brian just grumbled that he didn't know, they should do whatever the hell they wanted, and then abruptly left the room.

His reaction surprised me. I'd thought he was as desperate as I was for relief from hearing our mother's ceaseless nitpicking and humiliation of our father: *Why can't you stand up to Carl? . . . Don't come near me—you smell like those darn turkeys . . . What do I want with an ugly old cookie jar like that?*

Although I was sad for my father, I still thought he'd be better off without her. Maybe we all would have been. My mother's unhappiness oozed out in little cruelties that weren't exclusive to my father, and sometimes as warnings: *You kids make me so miserable. Don't ever get married and don't ever have kids!*

The truth was, I'd been complicit in my mother and Peter's affair. She'd surprised me by visiting on Parents' Weekend while I was still at the University of Wisconsin–Madison, but she'd had a hidden agenda.

During dinner at a local restaurant, she looked around surreptitiously and then giggled and said, "I'm seeing someone."

I'd grabbed that opportunity and said, "Well, I smoke cigarettes." If she could be a "naughty girl," so could I.

"I know. I found the Pond's cold cream jar full of butts under your bed after the last time you were home." She sighed. "Such a filthy habit. But Peter smokes too."

I pulled out a cigarette and lit up. That she was hurting my father bothered me, but it was only one more in a long line of hurts, and it teased the possibility that he might finally become free of her.

Then she asked me to have lunch with Peter and her the next time I was home, to see what I thought of him. Elevated to her co-conspirator, to someone whose opinion suddenly mattered, I agreed. A few weeks later, we snuck to a neighboring town for lunch. Peter was charming, and I had approved him. Such an easy mistake to make.

My mother dropped my father at one gate of LAX and picked up Peter at another. An efficiency of effort. Peter moved into our apartment building, while my father rented a room in an elderly woman's house in Illinois, instead of returning to our hometown in Wisconsin, probably to avoid the humiliation of having given up everything only to return home with nothing.

Only days later, my mother told Brian and me there wasn't enough money, and we had to move out and fend for ourselves. It was as if our family had fled our tiny hometown in order to implode in private. On top of having to cope with being extracted from our small town and dropped into a sprawling metropolis, Brian and I were cast out in the middle of a cultural revolution—it was 1967, the Summer of Love; sex, drugs, and rock and roll were the new religion, and our gurus, rock stars.

Brian soon lost his bearings, and years later, so did I.

Living in the Valley was like inhabiting a dollhouse world. Unreal, unalive. No mosquitoes and no flies, so almost no birds either. Only little trees, bushes. Instead of grass I could walk on, there was that ivy-type stuff—*pachysandra,* our grandmother said. Everything so *cute*—one-story ranches, the tiny yards sprouting gaudy orange and red and yellow flowers, the white rock "lawns," the blue pools. No history to the place—everything new, modern. No center to anything, no place to meet people serendipitously. Even the sidewalks, where they existed, were bare. No one walked anywhere. No downtown, only houses interrupted every now and then by a shopping center and crisscrossed by freeways like chains attempting to tie everything in place, but without much luck. Neighbors didn't seem to know each other, so I suspected people were transients, there for a year or two then gone. Houses had no basements, no attics, as if people knew there would be nothing worth storing, saving.

Nothing in LA reminded me of myself. I faded into the gray concrete of the streets and watched the make-believe world. I hadn't met a soul. I colored my hair blonde, thinking maybe my "colorless" hair (ashy light brown) was what had rendered me invisible. And now Brian and I would be on our own. Brian had graduated from high school right before the move, and except for my freshman year in a dorm, I had no experience living on my own or supporting myself. The only definite plan either of us had was enrollment at San Fernando Valley State in Northridge for the fall semester.

Brian arranged to share an apartment with Cliff, our cousin, while continuing to work at an electronics factory where he and my father had worked together for a few weeks, but soon he ditched what he called his "mind-numbing" job and found a new one in West Hollywood, parking cars at the Laurel Inn on Sunset Boulevard.

I convinced my mother to let me stay until September so I could save for an apartment. I reluctantly worked a few weeks as a not-very-good waitress at a Howard Johnson's, where I was yelled at by customers and cooks alike (and where I fainted twice from stress), and as a transcriber, typing videotaped conversations for a *Candid Camera* knockoff, a TV show canceled within days of my hire.

The transcriber job had fallen into my lap when I became so lonely I dared call Gary, a film editor, ten years older than I, and the cousin of a Wisconsin friend. He arranged the job for me, and even though it didn't last, we became lovers, and he introduced me to his Hollywood crowd. I was intimidated but determined to ignore my fears and inhibitions, try new things, and go with the flow.

I'd grown up an "all-American girl," president of my senior class, editor in chief of the yearbook, salutatorian, and at least until I went to college, had never touched cigarettes, alcohol, or drugs and was still virginal and a church attendee. Now I was whisked into a whirlwind of sex and drugs, of group sex, ice cube and whipped cream and leather belts sex; of parties at directors' houses where I sat mute among the sophisticated bikini set of Hollywood lovers and wives, who in turn sat watching the men swim in oddly shaped pools; or where everyone lounged around living rooms where mirrors were laid out with piles of cocaine, a razor blade for creating a line, and straws for sniffing.

At one of these parties, Gary and I dropped mescaline and while we were peaking, sniffed coke. When I noticed two guys playing Ping-Pong, I challenged the winner, and he rolled his eyes but agreed to a game. I held a paddle and served, and the ball flew low across the net, plinked the corner of the table, then flew off into the bushes. From then on, my serves were masterpieces of speed and strategy, my eye and arm floating exactly to where the ball was returned. I beat one man after another until they all wandered off. I smiled to myself. This was how life could be, should be—this glide of sureness, of victory.

At the end of the summer, I was still living with my mother. After the transcriber job fell through, I checked out job postings at Valley State and found a part-time clerical job for a small company that sold medical equipment (including, I discovered after I started, sexual prostheses and paraphernalia) via catalog. I also posted a ROOMMATE WANTED notice on a bulletin board in the college's cafeteria and found Judy, and we rented a two-bedroom apartment in Northridge, close to campus. I owned two pieces of furniture: a $10 mattress from the Salvation Army, which I plopped onto my bedroom floor, and a cedar chest my father had made for his mother when he was in high school, where I could store my clothes.

While the engine for the apartment complex's pool heater (unfortunately housed behind my bedroom wall) pounded in my head, I smoked cigarettes and wrote poems about holes and gray walls and stared at the sparkly ceilings, lost in the abyss, without hope. My mother had discarded me, tossed me away when she no longer needed me for bragging rights, for those articles about my achievements in the local paper that she could tout to her friends. Without family and friends, without the structure of familiar surroundings, I didn't quite know who I was anymore.

I decided if I couldn't be happy, at least I could make men happy. I bedded them, one after another, sometimes two in a day, and was brutally honest with them about everything—that I didn't care, that I hadn't had an orgasm, that it all meant nothing—because there was nothing to lose, since all was lost. It made me feel a little powerful, as if I were Tinker Bell freely granting them their wishes, except it felt a little soulless too.

Brian visited me and spied my birth control pills in my bathroom. He frowned. "So you're screwing someone?"

"I'm not 'screwing' anyone. I'm making men happy."

"Plural?"

"I'm not counting."

"So my father's a wimp, my mother's a witch, and now my older sister's a nymphomaniac. That's just groovy, man." He breathed heavily, fuming, almost snorting.

I laughed a little at that. "It's not like I'm enjoying it. And anyway, there's nothing wrong with it."

At least someone was touching me. At least I felt wanted. For something. I was aware of ignoring my conscience—it no longer seemed relevant. Everything was relative! A new world, free of outmoded ideas of morality! Do what feels good! Make love, not war!

One Saturday night that September, as a group of about ten people sat and talked and smoked grass, Judy and her boyfriend walked nude around the apartment, then settled into an armchair, and she gave him a blow job, while everyone pretended it was a perfectly normal expression of their affection. And it was—at parties, some people would always disrobe and walk casually around, clothes just another layer of superficiality, another layer of hang-up. Judy's friend Rocco got stoned and fucked a rose. *Wasn't that beautiful? So spiritual.*

I gained thirty pounds and for once had hefty breasts, D cup, compliments of the first batch of birth control pills. Maybe that was why I was so depressed, the hormones, but I felt as if my breasts simply expanded with each new lover.

I continued seeing Gary, too, and then went out with one of Gary's friends, then another. For the next year or so, my new friends and I immersed ourselves in the relentless screaming of acid rock, the melancholy of Ravi Shankar's sitar, the beating and booming and whining of music that pulled me down a tunnel inside my mind, the tunnel compliments of grass, hash, acid, mescaline, THC, psilocybin, belladonna, opium, peyote buttons. Served up in water pipes, carved pipes, metal pipes, spoons, capsules, slices, rolled in paper, cooked in brownies. I sat with other nameless people listening to live music (Cream, the Who, Janis Joplin, Blood, Sweat & Tears) or on the floor of someone's living room, stoned out of our minds, the music a tornado of sound around us, dipping our fingers into raw chocolate chip cookie dough, stupid smiles on our faces or fear in our eyes.

I didn't like the screaming music, the grass or hash—I felt lost in a void, obliterated by sound and feeling, unable to move or speak. The acid, the mescaline, made my insides grind with tension, my nerves taut with an energy so explosive I thought my whole body might burst into a million pieces. Some friends and I dropped capsules of dried and ground peyote buttons and built a dam in a stream, and when the water changed course, were rewarded with the revelation *Creation is destruction*. And we said to each other, "That's heavy, man."

But I loved the cocaine. At one party, another woman and I went outside, whisked off our shirts, and soared high on a pair of swings into a sky sprinkled with the few stars visible through the smog and lights, and I felt free and in love with the world and with Gary and even with myself, so ecstatic, such a feeling of well-being. I laughed and said to the woman swinging next to me, "I *want* to be addicted to cocaine." Of course, everyone *knew* it wasn't addictive.

Meanwhile, I excelled at Valley State. It was easy to get A's in California; I secretly thought all Californians, compared to Midwesterners, were educationally deprived. I could no longer count the number of people who had asked me whether Wisconsin was *on the beach*.

I worked at night, frightened to be in the dark building alone except for the maintenance crew, but I typed in the names, stuffed envelopes, and still had time to draw pictures, swirls of amoeba and angular flowers that I later taped on the walls of my bedroom, as well as time to type Brian's handwritten English compositions.

The first paper I typed shook me. My brother was supposedly brilliant, or so his teachers had told our mother, who made a point of telling me, humbling me with a little dose of implied "you're not quite as good," but his writing was like a fifth grader's, awkward and simplistic, with stilted phrases. Also didactic, as if he was driven to convince the reader of something of supreme importance, but the message was somehow hidden. I thought he wasn't putting enough energy into school, that he shouldn't be working full-time, but he wanted his own car so badly.

He bought a used black Austin-Healey convertible, was stopped repeatedly for speeding, lost his license, had it restored, earned more tickets and higher insurance costs, and complained, "Those fucking pigs, always picking on the little guy." He whipped other people's cars back and forth into parking spaces at the Laurel Inn, bought a hot watch from someone selling goods from the trunk of a car, was mugged in the lot, threatened with a knife, had his watch and class ring stolen, and started getting D's and F's at school.

I'd lived with Judy only a couple of months when my cousin Cliff called me.

"I come back from a weekend with Lily and I walk in the door and what looks like Brian's body is hanging from a rope in the archway. I was about to puke when Brian leaps out of his room, laughing like a goddamn hyena, and says something like, 'Pretty good joke, hey, man? Looks pretty real, doesn't it?' He'd stuffed his own clothes with pillows or socks or something."

"That's awful! Can you put him on the phone?"

"I yelled at him and he stormed out. I didn't think I should call your mom, but I thought I should tell someone at least."

Hours later, when I finally reached Brian, he said, "Cliff just can't take a joke. So friggin' uptight. It's a good thing he's moving out."

"Moving out? But what will you do?"

"I already found this really great guesthouse in North Hollywood, closer to work. And it's cheap."

"Isn't that too far from school?"

"I'm not doing too well. I need a break, man. They're just trying to make me think the same thoughts as everyone else—to make me a slave of the six or eight people at the top who decide what everyone should think."

"But you can't drop out. What about the draft?"

"Well, I sure as hell am not going to Vietnam! I already told Dad—fuck him, telling me I should fight for my country. What's this fucking country ever done for me, except to steal my money?"

What would he do next? Flee to Canada? Get arrested for draft evasion? "I'll ask around," I said. "I know some guys who are trying to get out of the draft."

After we hung up, I realized I'd forgotten to ask more about the hanging dummy, but I believed Brian enough to think the stunt was nothing more than a product of his twisted sense of humor, and, as my mother would have said, another bid for attention. It didn't occur to me to question whether it might imply an urge to hurt himself. He had a certain bravado that made him seem invincible, someone who would never consider something like that.

Brian had always been in trouble in one way or another: accidents, breaking bones, resisting, and rebelling, but he also seemed fearless in a way that was foreign to me, that I even admired. One night when he was fourteen or fifteen and our parents were out, he hopped into my father's pickup, told my friend Tess and me to climb into the back, and drove us to the drive-in movie theater thirty miles away. What a lark! It was thrilling to be an accomplice in breaking the rules.

But still I was afraid for him—dumped into this never-never land of concrete and anonymity directly from a country town. Still afraid for myself too. I was living paycheck to paycheck, unsure whether I'd be able to pay future tuition so I could continue with the only thing I was good at, achieving academically. And I had only one or maybe two semi-friends, no real safety net. The only option seemed to be to plod forward in spite of my depression, work hard, and hope for a grant or scholarship. It had paid off in the past.

Months later, after meeting with a psychiatrist I'd found, Brian was given a 4-F draft designation, meaning he was deemed unfit for military duty.

"I sure pulled one over on that guy," he laughed.

But I wasn't sure. We were sitting on pillows on the floor of the guesthouse he'd rented, smoking grass. He introduced me to his pet spider, Hazel. "Have you ever thought about how beautiful spiders are?"

I shook my head.

"Look how she creates her own home, pulls it right out of her own guts. Maybe Hazel's the reincarnation of a wise man, in my house to guide me, convey his wisdom."

"Why a wise *man*? Maybe it's a wise woman. What kind of wisdom?"

He was staring fixedly at his Jimi Hendrix poster and didn't answer, apparently mesmerized by the beauty of it all. It was an odd idea, but who knows wherein the truth lies? That type of metaphysical thinking seemed to be everywhere—people tossing coins and reading the *I Ching*, reading tarot cards, traveling to India to find gurus.

After one semester, I left Valley State, having discovered that LA Valley College, a junior college, cost only six dollars a semester. I sat in a philosophy class where one guy kept asking the instructor, "Does God do this? Did God really . . . ? What is life after death like?" As if the instructor had the answers and could simply tell that kid. That experience itself was worth at least six dollars. And I was captivated by an art history class, my first in-depth exposure to classical art, and I started sketching as I sat on the school's green lawns.

When I was about to become a state resident, I applied to UCLA and was not only accepted but also given a substantial financial aid package—a miracle! Why would UCLA want me? I was nothing but a body, raining happiness on other bodies, and an empty mind. My former achievements in high school and college seemed to belong to someone else. I was the girl whose mother laughed at her, told her she wasn't good enough, couldn't do anything right—*How can you be so stupid, Linda?*

Positive feedback, though, floated away like dandelion fluff scattered by any tiny burst of air.

How utterly surprised I'd been when Gary had pointed out my litany, "I'm so stupid," my default response to everything from bumping a table to genuine ignorance of anything, reflecting my own expectation that I should be as all-knowing as that junior college professor should have been, the inside info on God at his fingertips. Feeling inept was so ingrained in me, I wasn't even aware of continually calling myself stupid.

Without a car, I needed to live close to UCLA, so I quit my typing job, left Judy behind, and found an apartment above a garage in West LA with Wendy, the sister of a former lover. We painted a dozen wooden crates yellow, green, red, and orange, and stacked them in an irregular mass against the wall, then stuffed them with books and pictures and shells. I made orange and yellow burlap curtains and threw an Indian bedspread over an old love seat we rented from a student furniture exchange. An old cable spool, varnished, became an instant round table. A clay pot holding a sprouting avocado pit adorned its center.

I thought I might major in psychology, so once I was approved for work-study, I talked a UCLA psych professor into giving me a job as a lab assistant. For four hours a day, I sat in a six-foot square room, listening to the monotonous click of a memory drum as it slowly turned and exposed words to unwitting freshmen who I then asked to recall the list of words.

I went on a chocolate chip cookie dough diet, a half cup a day, until I'd lost twenty-five pounds. One morning I looked in the mirror and wondered where my breasts had gone. But at least I was thin again.

Brian went out with my roommate Wendy for a while, until he became too weird for her. I asked her if she knew what was bothering him, and she said that, among other things, he was worried about his penis being crooked when erect, that there was something wrong with him. "Not quite what I meant," I said, but immediately thought of the older boys in the Houston bathhouse years before, yanking Brian's penis (reportedly). A fledgling psychologist, I wondered what his worry might mean. Was he questioning his sexuality?

Settled in my new apartment, I invited Brian over for meat loaf, his favorite, and he told me about all the wonderful ideas he had for starting his own business and making millions. When he was young, friends and relatives said he'd probably make a lot of money someday, the way he worked so hard at his newspaper route, winning a bicycle, winning trips to see the Minnesota Twins. The way he hoarded his money, sitting for hours counting it in his room.

"Hey, look at these!" He smiled and handed me his sketches of clothes made out of hair—pants, shirts. "Human hair," he clarified. "So groovy! I already sent for patent materials."

I was mulling over the idea of "hair shirts"—some sort of metaphor? "Wouldn't they be itchy?"

"Nah," he said, grabbing for the drawings. "I also have plans for—get this—a jungle nightclub! You slide down a leafy tunnel to get inside. There'll be real jungle animals in cages inside, and a waterfall, and grass huts for dinner parties. So cool!"

"That *would* be cool—but, not to be a killjoy, where will you get the money?" I asked.

"Well, I know these people in the entertainment business, you know, from the Laurel Inn."

"Like who? Did they say they'd invest?" I didn't know—should I be talking him down or was there something to this?

"I've been invited to Tom Smothers's house—we're good friends actually, and another guy offered me a job as an extra in this movie. I'd be a cowboy. Maybe I'll be discovered, become an actor!"

"Wow, that would be so groovy!" Enough with challenging him—I didn't want to break his heart.

"My new friends are truer friends," he said quietly.

"What do you mean?"

"Remember when my old friends came to visit last month? They betrayed me."

"Which friends?"

"Denny and Jim? From Whittier? They stole my money and . . ."—Brian paused and sighed—"and Denny *killed* Hazel, my pet spider. Just stomped on her and wiped her onto an old newspaper. They didn't understand anything."

"That's terrible."

"I almost started crying, I was so frustrated, and I kicked them out. They weren't my true friends after all. Couldn't be trusted." He shook his head, looking tearful even now.

"I'm sorry about Hazel."

He seemed almost as distraught as when we were kids and his beloved dachshund Max was run over by a neighbor. He'd cried in his room for days. Inconsolable.

CHAPTER 2:

THE PROBLEM WITH BRIAN'S HAIR

I was worried about Brian. He was too isolated, and working as a parking attendant was a dead-end job, although he was occasionally rubbing shoulders with celebrities or at least exchanging keys with them. He seemed to think they might offer him some flashy, quick solution to what to do with his life. He was so lost.

I thought about calling my mother but knew she'd probably just deliver one of her usual rants about *how selfish* he was, and why couldn't he *just grow up and act normal*? When Brian was younger, our mother would often berate him, predicting he'd *never amount to anything*. Maybe he'd taken that to heart and was unknowingly acting out her expectations. Unless something changed, he didn't have a chance.

From an early age, Brian *had* been egotistical, self-centered, and often reckless and enraged. When we were in grade school, kids would run up to me and report: *Your brother just got beaten up by Eddie. Your brother's beating Benny up. Your brother's crying, and his nose is bleeding.* Not knowing what to do, I'd wince and avoid looking at where he was rolling in the dirt, socking someone in the belly, being punched back. I pretended it wasn't happening, that it had nothing to do with me. I felt both helpless and ashamed—of him and me.

Childhood photos of Brian revealed the scars of his battles: the half-inch slash near his left eye from the wild swing of little Jimmy's bat; the small bald spot visible through his crew cut, a scar from a board with the nail in it. Jimmy again? Or some other kid? Accident-prone, our parents said—had his accidental conception (according to my mother) been a portent? A broken arm from falling through the bulkhead onto the basement steps. Both wrists broken simultaneously in a careless jump. Broken fingers. And he'd had a few unusual medical problems: Almost dying from a bee sting. Surgery for ingrown toenails. At age four or five, he'd contracted scarlet fever and had a 106-degree fever, and the local doctor made a rare house call in the middle of the night to give him a possibly life-saving shot.

For years, Brian and I fought, socking each other, torturing each other with tickling or dangling saliva, swearing our hatred, how we wished the other were dead, but why so vehemently? Were we simply our mother's pawns, acting out her expressed wishes that we'd never been born? Our mom's pet phrase: *Why don't you just kill each other and get it over with?* Over for whom? When my father came home from work, she'd complain about our bad behavior, and he'd whip out his belt or grab the yardstick. One time he broke it over Brian's bare bottom.

But we hadn't always fought. When we were very young, we'd shared a bedroom, whispering nightly behind the toy cupboard that separated our twin beds, in the blue glow of our little lamb night-light. On hot summer nights, we slept in the swaybacked bed on the screened porch. In the morning, we played *Mess Up the Bed and Play Dead*—crumpling up the blankets and sheets, making canyons and mountains, and hiding tiny plastic cowboys in the canyons and caves, ready for ambush, for war with each other. Which of us had come up with the title for our madeup game? The theme song for our childhood already understood, our mother's unhappiness so palpable, translated in our childish minds to a wish for us to disappear. Such wisdom for a four-year-old, a five-year-old.

Brian was always sneering, laughing at authority. Being a smart aleck. Once he sat down at the counter of the Houston Café, and when Lovey, the waitress, approached him, he said, "A double maple walnut ice cream cone sure sounds good." When she returned with a tall, dripping cone, he said, "I didn't say I wanted one."

When he was a teenager, my mother told him to get down on his hands and knees and scrub all those filthy black marks from his boots off his bedroom floor. He filled a bucket with soapy water and went upstairs. I was lying on the sofa watching television in the den below when I noticed a discoloration on the ceiling that was spreading and wet. I hollered "Mom!" and ran upstairs. Brian had emptied the bucket onto his floor, and was on his knees in water, brushing at the black marks.

"How can you be so stupid?" Mom said. "You did that on purpose, didn't you? I know you did."

He looked back at her with an amused raise of his eyebrows. "I thought this was how you washed a floor, that's all."

How can you be so stupid? That oft-repeated phrase to both Brian and me. We, in turn, passed the message to our baby sister—*You're so stupid, Mandy*. Doing our mother's work for her.

When I had a friend from Whittier visiting overnight, my mother would suggest a prayer before supper. Inevitably, Brian would innocently ask why we had to say a prayer if it wasn't Sunday, and he'd smile slyly at me as our mother fumed. Or she might do something strange, like serve Jell-O salad on individual beds of lettuce, to make it *dressier*, but throwing the whole family into a state of confusion—and Brian would blurt, "Are we supposed to eat this lettuce or not?"

Such an egocentric kid. So conceited. Standing for ages in front of the bathroom mirror, wetting his hair, getting the front to stand up and form a *V* in the middle of his forehead. How he admired himself, but with reason—he was notably handsome, gorgeous eyes twinkling under thick, long lashes that I wished I'd inherited, a perfect nose (while mine was long, thin), a strong jaw. He had white, even teeth, while I'd needed braces to close the spaces.

But he was short. He grew to five foot two and then stuck there for years, smaller, powerless, picked on by taller boys. He must have been frustrated by his body, which might have partly explained his anger, which erupted so easily—red-faced fury if it looked like he wasn't going to win a game of Monopoly, although he usually did, the money whiz kid. Yelling at the television, raging, if his baseball team didn't win.

How he frustrated our mother, the church pianist, every Sunday morning, when she worried about getting to church. He would take his sweet old time getting dressed and combing his hair, while we all sat in the Pontiac waiting for him. My father would go back into the house and yell, but Brian just sauntered out of the house, a little smile on his handsome face, which triggered our mother's tirade: *Why are you so hateful, so selfish?*

Mom told me Brian's IQ was very high, even higher than mine, although he didn't perform as well; in his own words, he *didn't care to try*. But as he grew taller and more comfortable with himself, he gained some popularity in high school—it simply happened, while I struggled with self-consciousness and fear but managed to hover on the edge of the popular crowd because I was so nice, because to be otherwise was too frightening. Maybe I'd opened the path, an ice-cutter slowly creating a traversable expanse of ocean for the following ship, so that it was easier for him—at least in the outside world. People said, *He's got a lot going for him*. It was said about me too.

Then it was the early '60s and the Beatles, and Brian grew his hair—the worst thing he could ever do to our parents. The sole topic of conversation at the dinner table for years.

It was 1964, dinnertime, and I was staring at Dad's neck, sunburned and cragged like a dried-up creek bed, and trying not to hear. His huge hands were flat on the tabletop, his fingers white, as if barely controlling the urge to give Brian's head a good wallop.

"Why do you want to look like a goddamn girl? If you don't get your ass down to the barbershop, maybe we'll have to come in the night and cut it for you!"

Mom piped in, "You look like a hoodlum, a creep—why would you choose to look like that?"

"It's my friggin' hair! I'll wear it the way—"

Mom interrupted, "Why do you have to be such a good-for-nothing? Why can't you be normal? You're just like your crazy uncle Lewis—"

Lewis, our mother's brother, thought he was the next best thing to Eric Clapton and reportedly had persistent visions of the Virgin Mary standing at the foot of his bed.

"I'm nothing like him." Brian's face was red with fury.

"—and you'll probably end up in the nuthouse too. Maybe you're just not all there."

"This is bullshit!" Brian jumped to his feet.

"Shut your mouth, you impudent brat." Dad pushed his chair back.

Mom wrested control again. "What's wrong with you? Do you have a hole in your head?"

I couldn't stand it anymore, and jumped up and yelled, "Can't you ever just leave him alone?" and ran out the back door and sat on the top step, my back to the door and blocking the exit, the phrase *A hole in his head? A hole in his head?* bouncing around in my mind.

Brian's hair dipped across his forehead, didn't even hang over his shirt collar, but still it had been a source of outrage. Such a cool kid, daring to go to the dances at the Rainbow with the teenage strangers from Sylvan Grove. Picking up those pretty big-town girls, but not really "going with" any one of them.

Daring to drink and getting picked up for being drunk and disorderly, for fighting, while I dared nothing of the sort, stayed prim and proper and scared.

Even though he'd been excited about the move to California, he couldn't seem to find his footing when we were expelled from our home. At least I had my life as a student to ground me. But despite my worries, I didn't call my mother to talk about Brian. She was part of the problem.

CHAPTER 3:

BRIAN, LOST, 1968–1971

In the fall of 1968, I met Ian, another UCLA student, who was an aspiring writer, but for practical reasons, a business major. He had broad shoulders, a wide face, strong jaw, mustache, and twinkling eyes, and he exuded confidence, walking around campus wearing red sneakers, a sports coat, jeans, and a bowler. We were comfortable with each other and both loved literature and music. He drew me more deeply into art, theater, film, and politics. We were both against the Vietnam War, and for women's rights, civil rights.

We both loved camping—whenever we had a school vacation, we escaped the concrete and metal environs of LA to hike through redwood or sequoia forests, singing in harmony as we walked, holding hands, and sleeping tentless under the stars, waking up to blue jays squawking and raccoons walking across our sleeping bags. We drove to San Francisco, waved to the other VW Bugs and the VW Buses painted with peace signs and plastered with bumper stickers: PEACE NOW and MAKE LOVE, NOT WAR, and joined thousands of other protesters for anti-war marches. Back at UCLA, we walked out of class, protesting the firing of Angela Davis.

I cared about Ian. He was a good man, a rare find. Chemistry was mostly missing, but I thought it wouldn't matter that much. Maybe it was even a plus—he was interested in me, not only in my body, which I thought of as a foreign object accidentally connected to that part of me I identified with, my mind.

Ian moved in with me in the winter of 1968, and I suddenly had a social life, ready-made, with his friends and family. We visited his mom and stepfather almost every Sunday, more often than I liked—he was the oldest of three children, and a bit of a mama's boy, but at least I felt connected to someone or something. I didn't feel as though I myself had a family, except maybe for Brian.

Ian and I visited Brian in his latest guesthouse and could barely fit inside. It was about eight or ten feet square, but he denied feeling claustrophobic, said he didn't need much space, that people were greedy and thought they needed more than they did, that he just wanted to live the life of a common man.

Soon Brian quit his job and was crisscrossing the country, disappearing for weeks at a time. Periodically, he'd call: "I'm in jail in Las Vegas, picked up for vagrancy, and out of money. Can you wire me some?" Or, "I'm in Illinois, but can't get a job at Manpower until Monday, and I need just eight or ten bucks so I don't have to sleep under a bridge." And Ian and I ran out to the telegraph office and wired money, even though we were living on part-time incomes, loans, and grants.

Eventually Brian was back in LA, knocking on our door. As I made coffee, he told me he'd been down in San Diego, at the zoo, talking with the apes. "Those apes are pretty wise beings, people should realize."

"They talked to you?"

"Not out loud, okay?" He frowned, then tapped his temple. "You know, mind to mind."

"That would be cool, but . . ."

"Like there's this witch—I hate her—she makes me do things. She gets control of my mind—"

"What do you mean? How?"

"I don't know—electrical waves? Through the radio."

I looked out my kitchen window, wondering, *Am I the witch? Is my mother? Is he talking about a real person?* I was mulling this over while watching our neighbor Mrs. Perez feed her noisy chickens, incongruous but fun additions to our urban neighborhood.

"Hey, Linda!"

I looked back at him. He'd continued talking while I was distracted and was now a little annoyed.

"So can you do that? Make your head invisible?"

"What?"

"You have to stand in front of a mirror and concentrate really hard. Sometimes I can make my whole body disappear." Then he laughed. "A useful skill at times."

I called Mom.

"Brian isn't well. I think he needs help. Maybe if he could go back to school, he'd get focused on a real career instead of fantasy businesses."

My mother had married Peter, a quickie job in Las Vegas, and they'd bought a house in Chatsworth, not far from Granada Hills. "I wish we could help, but you know how Peter is. He thinks you kids should be able to make it on your own."

"What's Peter got to do with it?"

"If only Brian would give up that stupid car maybe he could afford school."

"I'm not sure he still has the car. But it's not about money, or not all anyway. He's a little *crazy* or something."

"Oh, he's just acting that way, trying to get attention like always."

"Isn't that crazy in and of itself?"

I hung up, angry at my mother's willful ignorance, her quick deflection to "how Peter is," as if she had no autonomy at all. Yes, Brian *was* attention-seeking—he needed help. But why did *I* have to be the one to parent him?

Brian visited Ian and me on my twenty-first birthday. He had a scab on his forehead, between his eyes. He said he'd been standing in a phone booth, fooling around with his jackknife, that it slipped, and he accidentally stabbed himself.

Later that evening, alone with me in the kitchen, he confided, "It didn't really slip. My hand just came up and shoved the knife into my forehead, and I couldn't stop it. It was like someone else was controlling my arm. It scared the crap out of me."

"But why would you—"

"I told you—it wasn't me!" He was agitated, grabbed his jacket.

I remembered another jackknife incident, back in Wisconsin. I was lying on my bed reading one day, when all the lights went out. I found Brian sitting on his bedroom floor, a jackknife in each hand. He said he'd just wanted to see what would happen if he stuck both jackknives in the outlet. He begged me not to tell our parents, and I agreed but told him not to do that ever again—it was dangerous.

Now he stared at me as he reached inside his jacket.

"Do you have it with you?" I held my hand out, thinking I should take it from him, but caught myself—he wasn't a child.

Instead, he pulled out a package.

"Happy birthday, from one fellow creature to another, even though you think I'm somehow an inferior mortal."

"I don't. I'm just worried . . ."

Removing the gift paper, I found two straw dolls. He was always giving gifts with messages. Voodoo dolls? A bit frightening, but I thanked him and asked where he'd found them—they were so unusual. "Some fair," he answered.

I picked up my tarot cards, which I'd been learning to interpret, and offered to do a reading for Brian, only to be terror-stricken when I turned over the card signifying death. I quickly faked the reading and piled up the cards, boxed them. Why couldn't they have come up with hopeful signs just this once?

Days later, Ian and I buried the dolls in the soft dirt under the trash barrel out back, both feeling silly but relieved.

I was taking an abnormal psychology class, finding symptoms of psychopathology in myself, but lots of students did—we joked about it after class. One day I walked into the elevator with the professor, and I told him there was something wrong with my brother.

"He seems to be paranoid schizophrenic, only no one believes it's real. They think he's acting, but isn't acting that way a form of mental illness itself? Do you have any ideas about what I might do to help?"

The professor backed up, raised his eyebrows, and looked away, as if I were the one who'd lost touch with reality. "I don't really know," he said, "and I don't make referrals."

His dismissal, his apparent aversion, surprised me. I knew people didn't usually talk openly about mental illness, but didn't he recognize me from class? Had he thought I might be talking about myself, not my brother? Now where could I turn?

That summer, my dad called and told me Brian had been hitch-hiking around Wisconsin, asking to stay with relatives and sponging off them. He said it was embarrassing and asked if I knew why he was acting so goofy. I didn't, but I said I'd talk to him. In a week, Ian and I would be driving to Wisconsin to visit my friend Connie in Whittier, a town north of Houston where Brian and I had gone to high school, and Brian was planning to meet us at her house.

Brian arrived grubby and disheveled, and asked Connie if he could shower. Later, when we were hanging out and smoking in my friend's yard, I asked him where he'd been staying.

"Here and there, wherever I find someone who cares more about a fellow mortal than how it's going to mess things up for them." Brian looked around my friend's yard, leaned over in his chair, and whispered in my ear. "I think I'm supposed to kill Aunt Bertie and Uncle Carl."

"What?" I jumped up from my lawn chair, and when Brian followed suit, I grabbed his arm and shook my head. "No!"

He wrenched his arm away, and his voice grew louder. "Yes—they made Dad weak, bossing him around in the turkey business, making Mom despise him. It's their fault."

I grasped his shoulders, shook him gently, and looked directly into his eyes. "No, Dad isn't really a weak person, and doing that wouldn't help anything. You'd just end up back in jail!"

Brian looked confused. "But—"

"You'd feel worse than you do already. Please, please, please! Promise me you won't do anything like that."

He again shrugged off my grip, looked at me sideways, shook his head as if disappointed in me, and walked away.

I told Ian I didn't know what to do. Was it a real threat? Should I warn my aunt and uncle, even though they lived hundreds of miles away? Or was it just talk? We decided the prospect of jail would deter him. We also didn't want to make his life even more difficult by notifying family or police over something that was likely just a passing idea. By the next morning he had disappeared again, back to California, we thought or at least hoped. Everyone was likely safe, but who knew? It took days before we relaxed and stopped asking whether we'd made the right call.

Months later, I invited Brian for Christmas and he arrived days too early. I was furious—I'd been studying nonstop for finals, hadn't showered in days, and wasn't prepared for the holidays—he simply couldn't stay. After he left, I berated myself. How could I do such a thing? Where was he sleeping?

But then I discovered he'd slept right below us—in the back room of the garage belonging to our landlord. He'd also rummaged around in the landlord's boxes and found an old goose-necked lamp and a can of silver spray paint. On Christmas morning, he presented me with the newly painted lamp, still wet, wrapped in newspaper. A message for me to "see the light"?

I gave him a set of acrylics, some small canvases, and a sketch pad, thinking it might help if he could express himself. He immediately started painting at the kitchen table, revealing himself to be an inadvertent pointillist, painting a long road into the mountains with tiny points defining the texture, the edges, as if his very self had dispersed into a mist.

Later that day, the three of us climbed into Ian's VW Bug and headed for Mom's house.

On the phone the day before, Mom had asked whether Brian would be coming, and I'd said yes.

She'd sighed. "If he starts acting weird, he'll just have to leave. Especially with all the relatives here. And you know how upset Peter gets with him."

"Mother—it's Christmas, and he's your son."

"It doesn't mean he gets to spoil it for everyone else."

It started out innocently enough. A little odd, the way Brian walked up to people, standing close, staring, and chuckling when they backed away. At the dinner table, Brian smiled and stared at the stuffed turkey for so long that Peter mumbled, but loud enough for all to hear, "What's he, on drugs or something?" And then even more loudly, "Brian, you want some or not? Spit it out, for Christ's sake."

Our mother said, "Just put some on his plate, Peter." She frowned a warning at Brian.

"I get turkey, huh?" Brian said, still smiling, staring now at his plate.

"You can have anything you want, you get a job." Peter downed his whiskey and soda, spread his arms, and braced his hands on the table. "If there's anything I hate it's a friggin' commie, excuse my language. Thinks everything comes for nothin'. A leech on society."

Brian struggled with his words. "Apes . . . are . . . noble . . . creatures."

We left the Christmas dinner early. I wanted to get Brian out of there before something worse happened.

I suggested to Ian that maybe we should let Brian come live with us. He needed a place to call home, someone to take care of him, and if Mom and Peter wouldn't let him live with them rent-free, couldn't he stay at our place? For a while, until he could get back on his feet? Ian agreed it was the right thing to do, and so we offered him a place to stay.

In one of my psychology courses, I was learning about behavior modification, which made me think that if Ian and I didn't reinforce Brian's irrational statements, if we just ignored them, maybe he'd *learn* not to say such strange things. Maybe insanity was just learned behavior, a way of adapting to a crazy world, and it was a crazy world, we all knew that. But this effort fizzled out quickly, when it felt more like we were simply ignoring *him*, not his words, since it seemed to have no effect.

A few days after moving in with us, Brian befriended a seemingly shiftless guy who lived in the neighborhood, with whom he smoked dope. He brought him into our apartment when we weren't home and gave him a loaf of bread and a dozen eggs.

"You can't just give away our food, Brian."

"He was hungry."

"Please don't bring him here again."

"You're just like all the rest, not caring about a fellow creature. We're all just a mass of atoms anyway, and now you're denying food to a fellow mass of atoms?" He shook his head in disgust and left. While afraid for him, I felt relief too.

I learned that Brian had wandered up north, when a minister in Oregon wrote me. While walking around a neighborhood in Eugene, my brother had followed a dog right into someone's house, thinking the dog wanted to show him something. Police escorted him to the state hospital, where he met the minister, who eventually invited him to stay in his home after he was discharged, until he felt ready to go back out into the world. The minister wrote that he and his wife had a little daughter who loved Brian. I was thankful that finally my brother had a family to take care of him, but I worried about the little girl, whether she would be safe.

But soon Brian was back in California, sitting on our sofa again, laughing, smelling of sickness, and with his hair chopped short—I wondered who had cut it. The hospital staff? The cops? Or Brian himself, trying too late to meet our parents' demands to cut his hair?

"You look tired or something," I said.

"Yeah, I'm not sleeping so well. Sometimes I'm so . . . I have these dreams . . ."

"What dreams? Do you remember them?" Maybe they'd provide clues to his illness. Maybe I could help him make sense of them.

"Like the other night . . . these big dogs chased me and tore me to shreds. And then I became a dog, too, and I was supposed to avenge myself, so I attacked them back and tore the flesh from their bones. I think I'm supposed to—"

Afraid to hear what he might say next, I jumped in, "You're not meant to act out your dreams. They aren't messages."

"But—"

"Usually they come from everyday experiences. Like the dogs next door that were barking last night. The dream just means you can do something about your problems, your fears."

"Like you friggin' know. They're *my* dreams."

I was scared. He was spending the night, and I was afraid to sleep, worried he might stab me, if he thought I was the witch he kept talking about, the one trying to control his mind, who made him have those terrifying dreams.

After a couple more nights with Ian and me, he disappeared again, then showed up at my father's, who had offered to share his small Illinois room with him. Dad tried to get him a job at the factory where he worked, but it didn't work out. Brian hit the road again to points unknown.

After a year and a half of living together, I suggested to Ian that we should get married. I thought of myself as jaded—I'd already seen everything, and he was that rarity, a good man. We bought simple gold bands, and I designed and sewed a red velvet wedding dress.

In June 1970, we drove to Big Sur and camped overnight. In the morning, I donned my red velvet dress in the wet-floored women's bathroom in front of curious campers, before Ian and I drove to a church in Monterey where we married in the garden, with two rough-looking landscapers (ex-cons?) as witnesses. I should have known when I'd accidentally, but irrevocably, sewed the velvet sleeves of my dress on backward that it was a sign. Or when we had to stop to buy a tie to replace the one Ian had, of course, forgotten.

I'd suggested marriage because I was afraid of the empty space that would otherwise be my future after graduation from UCLA. I loved him, but wasn't *in* love with him, and thought that would be enough. But I had second thoughts almost immediately.

With our apartment in LA sublet for the summer, we headed to a cottage we'd rented in Ojai, where sand from a nearby construction site blew through our screens and coated everything, where the ground was visible through holes in the bathroom floor. We didn't tell Brian where we were living, afraid he'd want to stay with us, afraid of *him*.

While Ian dabbled at working, selling almonds from his friend's farm stand, I commuted an hour each morning and night to a full-time job at Camarillo State Hospital. It was then I started suspecting our relationship might never be truly reciprocal, that I might end up taking care of him more than he could take care of me. I suggested having an open marriage and proposed that our interactions with others would just be sexual, not emotional, and might improve our relationship. It was common knowledge that no one person could meet all of their partner's needs. He agreed.

Ian came home unexpectedly early from work one day just as my lover Mark, a fellow research assistant at Camarillo, and I were leaving the cottage. He stomped toward us, his face red with fury. "You brought this asshole here? Why I should—"

"You're early—we were just—"

"Why'd you even want to get married?" He tugged at his wedding ring and threw it in the dirt at my feet, kicking up a little cloud of dust. "I'm not putting up with this shit."

"But you said . . . you agreed."

"Yeah, right, my fuckin' mistake." He elbowed me aside, stormed inside the cottage, and slammed the door.

Shaking, I picked up and pocketed his ring, and Mark and I left quickly on foot. What had I done? An open marriage was a mutual agreement to fool around, as long as there was no *emotional* involvement, as long as it was meaningless sex. But it turned out that it "meant" something, pain for both of us. I felt like a terrible person and wanted to run away from Ian and my own hurtful behavior.

That same day, Mark and I hitchhiked to Big Sur, where we stayed for a week or so, before going home to LA, where I just couldn't choose between them. I wished I could merge half of Ian with half of Mark to give me Ian's clever intellectualism, which challenged me, and Mark's stupendous sexuality, which made him harden just looking at me from across the room.

I wanted both of them and neither and ended up rejecting my lover, telling him over the phone please not to call again. Too much to give up—all my connectedness in LA was through Ian. When I imagined my life without him in it, I floated in empty space, untethered, inside the unreal. There was no world left, and I decided to opt for the world, for the familiar.

I slipped his ring back on his finger, and Ian and I settled back into our LA apartment and patched our relationship back together with little acts plucked from our past that had one time signified our love: me watching him from the window as he left for the day, tossing him kisses, the two of us cooking together, and Ian bringing me jars of fudge sauce for my ice cream.

A few months after we were back in LA, my father called and said Brian was in Minnesota, at Moose Lake State Hospital. He'd been ice-skating along a road, hitchhiking, and a guy in a pickup stopped for him. When the guy pulled over at a truck stop for coffee, Brian slid behind the wheel and drove away, apparently believing the man had given him his truck.

Now Brian was asking our father if he could ride with him to California for Christmas, a month away. Dad asked me what he should do. "Brian's acting so nutty—is he on drugs or something?"

"I don't really think drugs are the problem."

Drugs may have contributed to Brian's mental illness, but I didn't want my parents to think drug use explained his behavior. Drugs were too easy a scapegoat, a stand-in for something more complicated, and it let them off the hook.

I added, "And the hospital probably won't release him if they don't think the trip is a good idea."

That reassured my father enough to let Brian ride with him. When he arrived after dropping Brian off at Mom's, he stepped into our living room, grasped me in a bear hug, and kissed me. I was expecting the usual peck on the lips, but he began to slip his tongue into my mouth. I pushed him away, and whispered, "Dad, I'm your daughter!"

He let me go, said *hmm*, then immediately lay down on the couch and fell asleep. Hours later, he sat up. "Sorry for conking out like that. I didn't sleep the entire trip."

"Did something happen?" I asked.

"I let Brian take the wheel, but he was driving weirdly, so I took over again. And when we stopped to eat, he just kept staring at me and laughing. He scared the hell out of me. My own son. I didn't dare to sleep or let him drive. Didn't know what he might do."

Because of his lack of sleep, I attributed the tongue incident to mindless delirium.

A day later, Mom and Peter dropped Brian off at our place. He sat quietly in the living room with Dad and Ian, laughing to himself at times, and then walked into the kitchen and said to me, "Your hair is so long. You shouldn't ever cut it." And then he stared at me and said, "Is Brian coming for dinner?"

I looked back at him, searching for a hint of humor, and seeing none, asked, "Brian who?"

He looked perplexed, and hesitated, but finally said, "Brian Bailey."

I didn't know what to say, so I pretended it was a joke. "I thought he was already here."

I almost cried, watching him turn and scan the living room. Wanted to grab him and hug him and tell him to please come home from wherever he was.

Brian uneventfully returned to Minnesota with Dad, who dropped him off in the Twin Cities, where he said he had a job lined up. But he ended up in Moose Lake State Hospital again, before being transferred to Camarillo State Hospital in California—where nine months earlier I'd worked for the summer in the research department.

I didn't know whether to visit him at Camarillo or leave him alone. The family seemed the source of his problems. Maybe *I* was his problem, the older sister who never left him alone, who was always trying to suggest how he could better live his life—maybe I was the witch, not my mother. I'd seen the psychiatrist's report that supported his draft status, and it said Brian appeared "to confuse his own identity with that of his older sister." Maybe he'd improve without my interventions. I decided not to visit.

I was so busy anyway, working on my troubled marriage, analyzing data for my honors thesis, working part-time, and applying to graduate schools. I'd decided I wanted to study personality, not clinical psychology. I was more interested in the functioning of the "normal" mind, and anyway, I wasn't sure anyone could really help the mentally ill.

In May, after he was released from Camarillo, Brian went to stay with Mom, despite Peter's obvious aversion to him. I visited and was astounded. Brian seemed to be himself again—for the first time in years. He was getting his life together, attending barber school (belatedly complying with parental demands by cutting not only his own hair but others' too). And he was going back to work, he said.

"Why?" I asked. "Isn't that taking on a lot all at once?"

"I have to pay rent."

Later, I cornered my mother.

"You're forcing him to go to work so he can pay you rent? Can't you see that might be too much for him right now? So soon? On top of going to school?"

"Oh, he'll be fine as long as he takes his medication."

"It seems like a setup for failure."

A week or two later, Ian and I invited Brian to the grand opening of an art gallery. In the car, Ian asked how barber school was going.

Brian chuckled. "I accidentally cut a client's ear the other day."

"How badly?" I asked.

"Just a nick. I was a little worried about it, but so far they haven't kicked me out."

"They're probably used to students screwing up and snipping people once in a while," Ian said.

At the gallery, Brian walked around slowly, stiffly, avoiding people, wandering away right after we introduced him to friends.

I caught up to him. "How are you doing? Everything okay?"

"I just feel stupid in this old sports coat."

"It looks fine." Although I could see what he meant—it did look a little shabby.

"It's from the hospital's lost and found."

I wanted to cry.

A few weeks later, in mid-June, we invited Brian to a party we were hosting and picked him up at Mom's, since he didn't have a car or a driver's license. I hoped he might like one of the young women we'd invited. A relationship might be good for him. In the midst of the party, he looked awfully quiet, and I realized, too late, that maybe it wasn't a good idea for him to be in a situation where people were drinking and smoking dope. A little later, I looked for him, but he was gone. I thought he must have arranged a ride with someone else. I called Mom, but learned he hadn't arrived home.

The next day my mother called, and my heart sank.

"Brian's in LA County jail. He told the police he'd been hitchhiking when a man in a yellow Cadillac picked him up and started speeding. Brian said when the police flashed their lights and pulled the car over, he thought they were after *him*, so when the driver stepped out of the car, he slid behind the wheel and drove away. The little idiot. Grand theft auto, they said."

"Oh, my God. They're holding him?"

"No, they'll release him until his arraignment, whenever that is. Peter's going to pick him up."

Two days later, Brian called me. "Can you bring me some cigarettes?"

"You're still in jail? Wasn't Peter going to pick you up?"

"Yeah, but he couldn't make it yesterday."

"*Couldn't make it*? That bastard!"

Ian and I drove over, intending to take him home, but we were told he could only be released to a parent, even though he was twenty-two and an adult. But they wouldn't explain, so we just left the cigarettes.

I called my mother. "It's awful just leaving him there."

"It's his own darn fault—we can't run and rescue him every time he does some fool thing like that."

"Do you have any idea what goes on in those holding cells?"

"Maybe he'll learn his lesson then."

"You'd better get him a good lawyer, that's all I have to say," But then I muttered to myself, "You bitch."

It was the end of June 1971, and I had worked in the UCLA psych department for three years for various professors, but most recently was assisting with research related to personality testing. My own senior honors project was focused on sex stereotypes and sex role (double) standards, because of my interest in and commitment to the women's movement. I'd been accepted by UC Berkeley for graduate school in psychology, while Ian had been accepted by the MBA program at San Francisco State.

I was working on my honors thesis the night before it was due when Brian called from Mom's house.

"Everything okay?" I asked.

"Yeah, everything's fine. I just called to say hi."

"Hey, isn't your court date coming up soon?"

"Tomorrow . . . but I'm not worried about it."

"Mom and Peter got you a good lawyer then?"

"No, just, you know, whoever the court assigns or whatever."

"What?! They didn't hire someone?"

"It'll be okay."

"They're going with you to court, right?"

"No, they're leaving for Ohio. On vacation."

"How could they? Who's going with you?"

"Mandy said she and her boyfriend could take me."

"High school students? That's infuriating! Can I talk to Mom?"

"She's not here. No one's home."

"Listen, let me try to reach the ACLU, okay? Maybe they can help somehow. I'll call you back in a half hour or so."

"Sure, okay." He hesitated and then said, "Bye, Linda."

There was nothing the ACLU could do at the last minute, but their rep said if he was formally charged at the arraignment, they might be able to help.

I called Brian back, but the phone rang and rang and rang. Why didn't he answer? I thought about driving out to Granada Hills, but I was under deadline pressure, and apparently he'd gone out, so probably there was no point.

The next day I was at work when my mother called. "I don't know what to do. When we came home last night, all the lights in the house were on and all the doors had been flung open—Peter was pretty upset about that—and Brian wasn't anywhere."

"And he didn't come home?"

"No, and we're supposed to leave for Ohio today. Could he have gone to the courthouse on his own somehow?"

"He said Mandy was taking him."

"I told her to go to school when he didn't turn up this morning."

"Why don't I call the courthouse? I'll see what I can find out and call you right back."

Someone at the courthouse said Brian hadn't shown up for his court date, but that he'd been charged with a misdemeanor, not felony grand theft auto.

I called Mom back.

"That's a relief," she said, "the reduced charge. Why did he have to go running off like that again, though? He's done this so many times, just run off and disappeared, but still I don't know if we should leave or stay. What do you think?"

"You might as well leave." I knew Peter would be angry if they didn't, and maybe she was right that Brian had just run away again.

But a little later, I said to my coworkers, "I think my brother might have killed himself." It was just a feeling I had. A horrible feeling.

The next day, after a long bike ride to Hamburger Hamlet in Westwood for lunch, Ian and I rode home to see our landlady come bustling out of the house, saying the police had been there looking for me. My first thought was that Brian was in trouble again, but then Ian lifted the note taped to our door and quietly read it to me: "Your brother is dead. Please call 555-4536 as soon as possible."

I shivered and looked around helplessly. My breath caught in my throat, and I couldn't breathe for a moment. I didn't cry. It wasn't real. The police wouldn't write a note like that, would they?

Ian called the number while I sat on the couch, staring, my hands folded together in my lap, knees together. If I kept very still, maybe . . . *Please, God, let it just be a sick joke.*

And then Ian was sitting beside me, tears running down his cheeks.

"Why are you crying?" It seemed like he was acting, like we were in a play, only I'd forgotten the script.

"Some little kids found him. In a field a couple of blocks from your mother's house." He swallowed and took a deep breath. "He'd shot himself. In the head. With a rifle."

I sat still and thought a minute. "How do they know it's really him?"

Mom and Peter were on the road, not reachable, so Ian called my aunt Laura and uncle Bob, who lived near Mom and Peter. I heard him explaining, and then he nodded and said, "She's in shock, I think. We'll be there soon."

My aunt and uncle followed us to Magic Mountain, where Mandy, now seventeen, was working in an ice cream shop. We gathered in the manager's office and asked Mandy to sit.

"What's wrong? What's happened?"

"It's Brian," Laura said, patting her shoulder, and Mandy broke into sobs. I studied her, wondering at my own inability to cry.

Ian and my uncle Bob decided they'd identify the body. I insisted I wanted to go, but they said no, it would be too upsetting. Later I wished I had so I'd know for sure it was Brian, not someone who'd stolen his wallet and not some vagrant Brian had killed, planting his wallet on the body, so he could escape to a new life.

When Ian and Bob returned from the morgue, I asked, "What did he look like?"

Ian choked, then blurted, "He was hard to recognize."

"Are you sure it was him then?"

Ian was nodding yes. "His wallet . . ."

"Did he put the rifle in his mouth or to his temple?"

Ian coughed, and Bob jumped in. "His temple."

"The right temple?" I asked, searching his face.

Bob nodded, looking a little shaky too.

"Oh." It was important to have a picture in my mind of how it was.

CHAPTER 4:

BURIAL IN AN APPLE BOX, 1971

I leaned over the steering wheel, staring tensely into a blackness only weakly lit by the VW Bug's headlights, insects splattered all over the windshield. My foot lurched between gas and brakes when, from exhaustion, I fleetingly hallucinated deer jumping into our path from the grassy sides of the country road. I suspected the semi that had been barreling down on us for miles, threatening to rear-end us, was part of the Olafson Transfer fleet, and that Ole himself might be at the wheel, annoyed by this out-of-stater, not realizing it was none other than twenty-three-year-old Linda Bailey from his own hometown, Houston.

Ian slept in the reclined passenger seat, leaving Mandy only a cramped space, but she'd managed to stretch out across the back seat. Sweat rolled down my forehead into my eyes, and my skin felt grimy from the dust of the narrow country road. We'd been driving nonstop for over twenty-four hours, heading back to Wisconsin for Brian's funeral, and I was afraid of falling asleep, despite the air blowing in the window. My shoulders ached, and I debated waking Ian to take a shift, but there was no place to pull over anyway, just a ditch on either side of us, with tall grass drooping onto the crumbling blacktop. I laughed quietly, but a little hysterically.

"What's funny?" Mandy whispered.

"The accident sandwich we're in—imaginary deer ahead and that semi climbing up my ass."

"Pull over—you're losing it!"

"Fat chance, baby sister—there's no room."

I wondered if life had felt like that for Brian—no way forward, imagined obstacles ahead and only threats from behind. Throwing those doors open, turning on all the lights in the house—hadn't that been his suicide note? That now he would be free? Even joyfully free? Or, more disturbing, could it have been accusatory, that now we could be free of him?

I wondered if my father was at this very moment looking down from a plane far above us, having flown to LA to escort Brian's body back to our hometown for burial. Mom and Peter were heading in their camper up to Houston from whatever town they'd reached before being pulled over due to an APB, the family now converging in Houston after flying apart in a kind of entropy four years earlier.

It was strange being in Houston. Everyone so happy to see us, as if Brian's death was just an excuse to visit. People wanting to take our pictures, chatting about their families, being so unfailingly kind, as if I could listen or care, when all I could think about was the horror of what had happened.

We drove past the old pool hall, with its Western facade and peeling paint, where on hot Sunday afternoons, I used to hang out with one or two other teenagers, the main street of Houston bereft of cars, none parked, none passing through. I'd thought I might never make it out—the sticky black tar of the pavement might permanently glue my bare feet to that dead street, melt them down to stumps, and I would stand there forever like a statue, waiting for something to happen.

The funeral home overlooked the Houston pond where Brian and I had swum and skated as kids. When Ian parked in front, Anson Milward, the funeral director, rushed over and leaned through my open window and, with an incongruous smile, spouted a welcome that seemed bizarre, as if it were a joyous occasion, as if thanking us for our business. I reflexively jerked away, but Ian leaned over and rescued the awkward moment with a little meaningless chatting of his own.

Once recovered, I climbed out of the car and stepped gingerly toward the door of the funeral home, tailing Ian and Mandy. Stopping at the entry, I saw the casket and then an old boyfriend sitting reverently in a chair, his head bowed, and I quickly turned and lurched back to the car, hysterical, whining, "No, no, no," but weirdly tearless—I couldn't seem to cry, as if my tears were frozen inside of me.

Later, I sat in the funeral parlor wearing a short flowered dress, unstockinged, my almost waist-length hair shadowing my face. I didn't have funeral clothes, but what did it matter? I listened to the red-haired kid, Alan, singing a song, watched Brian's high school friends lined up along the side wall, the pallbearers, and imagined Brian sitting on top of the casket laughing at us, laughing at us all, just like when he was a kid—always getting the last word, winning that way. And I started laughing to myself. All the hypocrites sitting there crying, people who ignored him, chose not to help, when he was alive. My mother sitting in front of me, sobbing, but one hand primping her hair. I quietly laughed again, imagined tears running down my own cheeks, wiped at them, and then rubbed my dry fingers together.

When we were finally at the cemetery, awaiting everyone to assemble, I steered Ian away from the relatives, the so-called friends, the so-called people who cared, who I heard whispering: . . . *heard it was drugs, probably that marijuana or LSD or some such . . . could've been murdered, no one's saying . . . he was talking funny, maybe he was in a cult or something . . . always asking for trouble, his poor folks . . . such a smart kid . . . such a smart aleck . . . had a crush on him forever, if only . . .*

I shook my head and lit up, smoking one cigarette after another, and snuck one to Mandy, who looked lost, hugging herself as if she were cold, despite the unbearable heat. I was comforted to see that Brian's plot was with our grandfather's.

I said to Mandy, "Do you think Brian would be peeved about the flat stone we ordered? And the simple service at the funeral home?" I had advised my dad about both, and now I wondered why. Why so discreet? It felt now like an attempt to sneak his death past everyone, keep it our dirty little secret.

"Maybe. He'd probably want a big one like Roger's down the row—with his picture on it."

"Yes. He'd want a big fucking stone." We both chuckled a little.

When the service was over, just before they lowered the casket, when everyone was drifting back to their regular lives, I walked up to the casket, laid my hand on it—the last one to touch him in this life. Just then I heard a dog bark and looked around to pinpoint the source, but saw none. I shivered, as if it were a sign, Brian signaling me. Maybe it was his dachshund Max welcoming him? A happy thought weirdly flying up through the gloom.

Mom and Peter continued on their trip to Ohio, which I found unfathomable. Back in Granada Hills, Mandy and I packed the meager remnants of Brian's life (drawings, writings, letters, photos, yearbook, wallet) into an old apple box, a Red Delicious apple on its side, and labeled it "Brian's Things." Ian and I carted it to our apartment, saving my mother from perhaps disturbing discoveries, like his essay on *The Witch*. And simultaneously, hiding from others and myself any evidence that might support my own guilt.

PART II:

THE BERKELEY YEARS AND BEYOND, 1973–1981

CHAPTER 5:

BELONGING, BE LONELY; ALONE, BE LONGING

Right after the funeral, Ian and I had to find an apartment in Berkeley and then pack and move before starting classes. I'd been given a job as a teaching assistant for an intro psych class and was terrified—there was no guidance about how to lead discussion sections, and I spent endless hours preparing. There was barely time to eat or sleep, much less to grasp what my brother's death meant to me.

Awash with new friends and demanding work our first year in Berkeley, Ian and I had little time to pay attention to each other. We entertained friends, cooked dinner together, and sometimes he brought me flowers, but we also went out separately with our own friends, male and female, while periodically threatening to leave each other. A year later, I bought a bestseller, *Open Marriage*, and proposed we try that lifestyle again, and Ian once again agreed.

I was besotted, smitten, with Matthew, a former professor of mine, who was witty, brilliant, and just plain fun. For a couple of months, we shared laughter and stimulating conversations over late afternoon glasses of wine, but it ended one afternoon when he called and said he was *too middle-class for this relationship*. Although too devastated to ask what he meant, I supposed it was that I was married. Before he left the area, he offered me a consolation prize—telling me I'd been one of his best students ever, neatly tucking me back into my role as former student.

The affair reminded me of what was missing in my marriage. Even though Ian and I had mutually agreed on an open marriage before my first affair, he hadn't taken advantage of the opportunity. This time, he did, but only half-heartedly. He saw someone once or twice, but it felt more like he was aiming for parity with me, not that he desired her. The open marriage concept had its flaws. For one, I still felt guilty, and for another, it was never just about sex. I was looking for a relationship that was mutual in all important respects. It occurred to me the lack of chemistry between Ian and me might be mutual. He might love me, but I suspected he wasn't in love either, that instead, he needed me more than he wanted me. I hated feeling needed. I wanted to be wanted.

But it was more than just a lack of chemistry. Ian was sometimes pompous, "holding forth," as I thought of it, hogging the limelight among friends. And he wasn't always good to me. Calling me *monkey-tits* because my fashionably thin body came with deflated breasts. Punching the wall and breaking plaster or ripping his own shirt when he was frustrated or angry. Once when we'd talked tentatively about splitting up, he'd told me I was *vain for no good reason*, *immoral*, and worst of all, *vapid*, and no one else would ever love me. Although apparently, I wasn't so awful that he was happy to let me go.

Brian's suicide had, for a while, knitted us together in the hug of tragedy. But now, whenever I looked at Ian, I was reminded of those years of Brian's decline into paranoid schizophrenia, how Ian knew the ways in which I had failed Brian and had seen firsthand the wreckage that was Brian's lifeless body. How would I ever be able to move forward if I stayed with Ian? I'd never really grieved Brian. Leaving Ian might give me that breathing space.

In 1973, two years after Brian's death, I rented a beautiful redwood cottage situated in the midst of trees and flowers, a garden of Eden in residential Berkeley, within walking distance of the university, the supermarket, the laundromat. I'd convinced Ian I needed to try living alone, being independent, just on a temporary basis. But I suspected that my dread at the sound of the little bell on his key ring signaling his arrival home at the end of the day was telling me we just weren't right for each other.

I'd come to feel a little like Ian's mother, reminding him of things, finding things he misplaced, taking care of stuff. Or like his sister—we were good friends, but not much more. In a strange coincidence, the day I moved out, Mother's Day, my father-in-law, ignorant of my plans, called to thank me for being such a wonderful "mother" to Ian, saying I'd been such a good influence on him, getting him to perform in school. I hadn't actually played much of a role, except possibly by example or in nudging him once in a while.

I still wasn't 100 percent sure moving out was the right decision, but as I told my friends, I'd felt the urge to leave more and more frequently, and how often do people ever reach a point of certainty about anything? Decisions were so often a crapshoot, but people usually found a way to justify them, to live with themselves. I guessed I would too.

My redwood cottage was conveniently within walking distance of the liquor store, and by September, I'd already trod that particular mile, carrying two gallons of red wine, five days' worth, too many times to count. I was beginning my third year in graduate school, and having earned outstanding evaluations, I'd been given a Regents' Fellowship, so I didn't need to work.

I had few classes and just needed to write my master's thesis, now that I'd collected all my research data. There was no place I had to be, and time slowed, opened up, tried to gulp me. I, in turn, guzzled my cheap red wine.

Leaving Ian, living alone, had started out okay. Decorating, hanging prints on the wall, buying a saw and making shelves for the bathroom, fixing beef stroganoff for one or inviting friends to dinner. Such freedom, just myself to care for. I went to an occasional party, went cross-country skiing and snow camping in Yosemite with a few friends (the warmth sucked out of my body until I thought I would die if I fell asleep), had a few lovers, had coffee with friends once in a while.

But gradually my life outside of home contracted, until I no longer roamed the campus or the city. Over a period of months, I took my independence to an extreme, until I no longer suggested movies or dinners out with friends because I lacked a car and would have to ask them to pick me up. I ultimately felt not quite up to entertaining—I alone wasn't amusing enough; Ian had been the star at all our dinners. I refused to call people. It would imply loneliness, neediness, and I wanted to be free of need, any kind of dependence.

Even in the cottage, I gradually spent most of my time in the bedroom, eating and working on my bed, locking even my bedroom door against the world. When I had to leave my apartment, for a class, for groceries, for wine, I felt a bit frightened, self-conscious, exposed. As if I didn't belong anywhere but in that redwood bedroom. When I came home, I couldn't resist checking the closets and behind the translucent door of the shower, nonsensically afraid of someone hiding or of finding a dead body hanging there, blood dripping.

I wrote a little poem, which I thought captured the paradox of my whole life:

Belonging, be lonely
Alone, be longing.

When I was inside a relationship, a role, all I wanted was out—I felt I had to yield too much of my *self*. When I was finally outside, I wanted to be in; a part of my *self* was missing.

One afternoon, after a seminar, I walked across campus with my advisor, a Renaissance man, broadly knowledgeable, not just stuck in a little academic niche like some other professors, who seemed to me to be weirdly eccentric and half dead, removed from everyday reality.

He commented, "You seem so forlorn—is it the separation?"

I looked up at him, his somehow charming underbite, humbling in its imperfection, his warm eyes, and then looked down, thinking. I wasn't certain why I felt so depressed, so aimless, but still I whispered, "I had a brother. He killed himself, blew his brains out the summer before I came here." I hadn't told anyone until then, so ashamed I was—my family, my life so alien, outside the norm.

"What a tragedy," he said, but looked away and said no more. I felt confirmed—it wasn't something that could be talked about. I must hoard my secret, keep it from the light, cut off that part of myself, remake history, pretend I'd never had a brother.

I met Ian for breakfast or drinks once in a while and helped him move into an apartment in San Francisco. Sometimes he visited and we had sex, but I felt guilty for hurting him and also vulnerable in that exposed position—that he might want to hurt me back. Once I imagined him plunging a knife in my vagina. But I still cared about him and was afraid to let go, worried about what he might do to himself—because I had missed the cues before, with Brian.

A few months after Ian's move, when finally he seemed to be doing well, I admitted over the phone that I wouldn't be coming back to him.

He flew into a rage. "You lied, you lied, and I could kill you for that! I'm going to come over and kill you, goddamn it all, you are such a lying bitch!"

Wrong yet again. I'd worried he might kill himself, when the danger was that he might kill *me*. Where could I hide? In the closet with the imagined hanging body? Maybe I could prop a chair against my only door. The locks surely wouldn't be sufficient to keep him out. But the windows—he only had to break one. Nowhere to hide, not really. Should I call the police? But maybe he didn't mean it. Probably he didn't.

And he hadn't come after all, and finally I slept. The next day, I contacted a lawyer. There was such a thing as clarity after all.

Free of Ian, I was still firmly invested in not needing anyone else either, but found myself drowning in alcohol. I hadn't considered that physical dependence might be inconsistent with my mission. And what exactly was this so-called mission? To determine the meaning of my life? To be free of all need? How many days, weeks, had I sat on the bed in that redwood cottage, smoking, drinking, listening to music, trying so hard to arrive at some understanding of my life? Alone. Believing I must be alone to work it out. Drawing pictures that repulsed me, writing whiny, maudlin entries in my journal, along with some very bad poetry. Spilling wine on my drawings, tearing them up, passing out.

The blackouts frightened me. Once I awoke in late afternoon to find a Carole King album lying on a pillow on the floor, as if it were a crown jewel, and couldn't recall bringing it into the bedroom or why—the stereo was in the living room. I looked closely at the album—it was the one with "Brother, Brother" on it. Had I been thinking about him? A message from my unconscious to myself? Had Brian come in ghostly form and transported it there?

Another time, I found the phone off the hook when I'd been awaiting a call from a man I'd flirted with all evening at a rare outing, a dinner party.

Once I found myself nude, standing over the trash container, urinating into it, as if everything in me was trash.

Another incident. I discovered all my clothes in the cedar chest were wet, though odorless, as if I'd deliberately poured water on them or—I was horror-stricken—urinated on them, mistaking the cedar chest for the toilet in my alcoholic stupor. The cedar chest my dad had made for his own mother, the one I'd spirited away for my apartment in LA, my "hope chest," the one that looked like a coffin sitting at the foot of my bed. I'd made the apartment, my bedroom, a coffin where no one lived, just the ghost of a person, a haze of smoke.

Then there were the illnesses, the gastritis from drinking, so that I couldn't keep food inside me. Walking across campus, praying for the continued tightness of my sphincter. Wine, then Maalox. Wine, then Kaopectate. The bronchitis that terrified me, that wouldn't go away, that kept me sitting up in bed for weeks, my breaths shallow, coming from my throat, as if my lungs were filled—I was going to die, I knew I was, and nobody would know or find me. I lay in bed, weepy, listening to the love songs on the radio, trying to swallow the wine, but it was so hard with the lump in my throat.

I visited a doctor, sure I had throat cancer.

"My only relief from the lump is wine."

"How much do you drink?"

"Two gallons a week maybe." More like three.

"You're young—why are you drinking so heavily?"

"Worry about orals, I suppose."

But I didn't tell him the rest: How could I go to sleep at night? Wine. How could I dare to go out in the world? Wine. How did I get to my inmost being? Wine, the only way—it loosened me up, freed me to be myself. The door to something real inside me.

Not that anyone knew. Well, now this doctor did. But he couldn't find anything that would account for the lump in my throat.

Before I left, he asked for my phone number, and I handed it to him (he was attractive, not much older). But then I casually asked, "Is that okay? Is it professional?" Inadvertently ensuring he wouldn't call.

I made it to my occasional classes and an occasional party. At one party, my friend Carol told me she liked me better when I was a little bit drunk. I liked myself better that way too—not so uptight, so worried. I was wittier when I drank, flirtatious, free from anxiety. The life of the party, in fact. Dancing, dancing, coaxing people onto the floor for circle dances.

Over a period of a month or two I wrote my master's thesis while sitting on my bed, gulping coffee, smoking, and for a while feeling okay, even excited. I wrote up the results of my research on the phenomenological experience of control (the attribution of responsibility for occurrences to others or to self—internal vs. external control) but took it further until I was lost in it, had developed a whole theory of personality. I sat on the bed overcome with the excitement of discovery, of having identified some form of truth in the way people experienced their own behavior. This was what Freud must have felt, I laughed to myself.

My advisor said it was one of the two best master's theses that ever came out of the department (I wondered who wrote the other one, and when). He suggested I should do research on different aspects of my theory and submit pieces of it for publication—the scope of it would keep me busy for years. But I thought, *Why should I? Let someone else do that.* What I liked was developing the theory. And research never quite captured the truth of behavior, of the individual life. Maybe only art or writing could.

1974. Post-thesis depression had set in. Pre-orals panic. Overwhelmed with my aloneness, with my anxiety, I thought I might be losing my mind. I panicked, believing the professors who praised me would discover the void within me, that I didn't know anything. One had said I was capable of making a significant contribution to the field (contributing my brain to the field of psychology, while my brother donated his gray matter to a more concrete, yellow grassy field, I couldn't help thinking), but my major problem was that I didn't know it. Another had once called me a *genius*—when I laughed and challenged him, he insisted he wasn't being facetious.

I had graduated from UCLA with psych honors, Phi Beta Kappa, and a published journal article, and was excelling in grad school but still felt like an impostor. I had merely given the illusion of intelligence and depth, of knowledge, through a certain intensity, a seriousness, that I created by frowning slightly and squinting my eyes. When the pretense was lost, there would be nothing left. My advisor was wrong, so wrong, when he said I could pass orals without even studying. I could see myself blocking, sitting in that chair in front of the committee, my mind drained of all thought, my tongue and lips paralyzed, my eyes crossing in fear.

It had happened before, standing in front of a group of undergraduates, leading a discussion section when I was a teaching assistant. My mind suddenly blank, struggling to remember what was asked, what the answer might be, frozen in place, time standing still, the students looking back and forth, wondering, *What's wrong with her?*

Besides, I couldn't imagine following through with this career, couldn't see myself standing in a lecture hall, the discussion group multiplied by tens, a whole roomful of undergraduates whispering, evaluating me, joking about me. Couldn't picture myself among some of those professors in the department, crazier than the patients in the clinic, one of them wearing plastic bags over his shoes when he walked into his lab, others studying little broken-off pieces of human behavior in tiny offices, and then writing obscure research papers about these toenail clippings of life that nobody really wanted to read. But what about the big picture? Life? The meaning of? The experience of?

I was drunk, alone, afraid I was going mad, smothered with fear, and empty of hope, and it didn't matter to anyone what

I did with my life, whether I lived or died. Maybe if I drank a gallon of wine all at once, then swallowed a bottle of aspirin, I would just die, put an end to my misery, my self-disgust.

Was that what Brian had felt? I imagined him sitting in that yellowed field with the rifle, possibly for many hours, no longer despairing, but still lingering, remembering a few good times, a last-minute check on whether it was the right thing to do, then concluding yes, and laughing—he had lost his mind and couldn't get it back. He bowed to his imagined audience, and then, emptying his head of all thought, pulled the trigger. I could picture the red and gray matter scattered over the dry yellow grass, the little boys finding him, their screams.

My head swirling with dizziness, a late afternoon yellow light making me nauseated, I dialed a friend, another graduate student, and begged him to come over. I was afraid I was going to kill myself, I said. He *tsk*ed, disgusted with my self-pity, as I was—another reason just to do it—but he couldn't come right then, and said maybe I should call 911.

I ran from the house, wandered drunkenly to a park down the street, waded in a tree-bowered stream, no one there, stepping on ice-cold wet rocks, from rock to rock. What was I doing? What was wrong with me? The cold wetness calmed me, awoke me from my drunkenness, and I trudged back. Nowhere else to go but home.

And there my friend was, with his girlfriend, waiting for me, worried. I was struck with a new wave of self-disgust; I was such a mess, piteous, all the neediness I abhorred on display, all my independence down the drain. They sat with me until I insisted I was okay and gave me the name of a therapist I should see.

I burst into tears when I first sat down with the therapist. "I think I'm an alcoholic, and I just feel like killing myself."

The therapist frowned slightly, leaned back, her fingertips together, and said, "Maybe I'm not the person to help you then. Maybe you should be hospitalized."

Hospitalized? I felt slapped. What kind of therapist would say a thing like that? I wasn't *that* sick.

I countered, "Suicide isn't a true option—it's already been done—my brother. Two suicides in one family—that would be a double whammy to my parents, and I don't want to hurt them quite that much."

"So tell me more about what's going on."

A man I didn't know well, but who worked in a neighboring department, started flirting with me. I'd never paid attention to him before, as he seemed a bit of a buffoon, but I was so lonely I responded a bit, and then he accelerated his campaign. He just happened to be my therapist's husband, and somehow, in my despair, his attention seemed like part of an organized effort to take care of me. What difference did anything make anyway? So I allowed him into my bed.

When a friend, who somehow found out, remarked that if I'd sleep with him, I'd sleep with anyone, I wondered, a little too late, how I could ever show my face in the department again. He started to leave me love notes in my department mailbox, while I tried to ignore him and the mess I'd made. When he told his wife, my therapist, she called me and demanded that I come see her immediately, saying that she *thought something like this might happen.* Which I thought was an odd thing for her to say—because of her husband? Or me? I never went back. I didn't need to add her anger to my self-disgust. I was my own best critic.

CHAPTER 6:

THE LOVELY LURE OF ENTRAPMENT

October 1974. Realizing I was too isolated, I pulled myself together long enough to find a living situation with other people. My friends Dannie and Eric and I found a brown-shingle house and then interviewed for one more roommate, choosing a house painter, Jake, to join our household.

The first time Jake and I were together—first kiss, first sex—was the night of the Halloween party my roommates and I threw. Jake had initially dressed in a Chinese robe until I convinced him it was racist, next in a silver leotard as Rudolf Nureyev (too revealing), and finally as a pirate—the perfect costume alighting last in his mind. He'd already extracted one of the two mattresses on my bed and borrowed my sheets, my towels, as if he had just as much right to them as I did. Good doobie that I was, I sewed myself a Robin Hood costume out of green felt, complete with quiver and cardboard arrows for threatening the rich so I could give their goods to the poor. So there we were, Robin Hood and the Pirate, two unlikely candidates for love but both thieves ultimately.

Jake the Pirate said he didn't believe I was an alcoholic when I declined a glass of wine and told him why, that I hadn't had a drink in a month (after several failed attempts to stop, which I didn't mention). That was all I needed to decide maybe I could drink after all. Maybe my drinking had been out of control because I'd been depressed and alone, but I wasn't anymore. Anyway, the party would be much more fun if I was a little bit drunk.

Jake was gorgeous—tall, slender, with thick longish black hair, a black handlebar mustache, dark skin (compliments of his Sicilian ancestry), and beautiful white teeth. When I saw him playfully nuzzling our roommate Dannie on the front porch (pirate snags beautiful dame), Dannie a knockout in a come-hither satin slip that skimmed her body, I decided I wanted him for myself—Dannie had a boyfriend anyway. I flung the door open, grabbed his arm, and pulled him into the house and onto the dance floor, where we danced wildly and sang along with what we both thought was Linda Ronstadt's "You're So Good," only to discover weeks later the title was "You're No Good"—an early and prescient (but ignored) warning that he wouldn't be good *for me*, at least.

I should have known by his wink the day he moved in. Never trust a winker—male or female, for that matter. Even then, before the party, I felt an inkling of disgust, a warning shudder at his condescension. When he left to run an errand, Dannie and I had snuck into his room, giddy with our daring. Our laughter was stopped short by the only decoration in his room—a calendar with a topless woman straddling a Moto Guzzi—which he hung because of the motorcycle, he later said. Why hadn't I believed him then? Was it any better to discover that he found women a poor second to that sexual machine, the motorcycle, than to simply let my feminism go down the tubes with winks and nudes in order to allow the relationship to happen at all? Still, I later hopped on that bike and rode, sitting behind him, covered in helmet, jacket, jeans, and boots, unable to speak, the wind and engine sounds roaring in my ears, drowning out everything. An escape, hidden in the noise of nothingness, hidden in his shadow.

I was startled when, the morning after the party, he hadn't disappeared, but instead pulled me onto his lap, an instant couple. He soon moved into my bedroom, and a new roommate moved into his.

For our first Christmas together, I made him a green velour robe, soft and plush, and a suede portfolio to hold his poems. And I had written a poem to enclose, with the first lines: *You take me home again, to warm kitchens.* Why hadn't that sounded the red alert? Why hadn't his poem "Excremental Awe" sent me running, the man standing nude, shitting in a garden, *on* the garden, and glorifying it—his shit as gold? Instead, Jake and I spent all our free time together, gradually retreating from our roommates and shared spaces to our bedroom.

Even as Jake and I professed our love for each other, I wrote poems about the meaninglessness of life, goodbye letters to friends, and a will, preliminary to my own imagined suicide. Not that I had a specific plan (notwithstanding my inane drunken attempt a few months before, making Sominex pancakes too disgusting to eat), but I had sunk deeply into a familiar depression, unable to see a way forward. I felt as if I were living simultaneously on two different paths—a simple life of love with Jake and the imagined relief of death, as if they were somehow comparable.

I worked on my personality theory at my desk, while Jake watched me, his eyes drawing me to the bed, his mouth saying, *Of course, I don't mind you working.* But what was I doing here? I was still terrified of taking my orals—I would be discovered as the know-nothing I truly was. And was this career even one I wanted? Was it worth this stress? I still couldn't envision myself as a professor, standing in front of a room of smirking or bored students, and the ability to do psych research seemed inexorably linked with academia. But if I left school and gave up my fellowship, I would have no immediate way of supporting myself.

Even so, on Brian's birthday, I dropped out of school. Academia wasn't real life. The last time I'd put my career first, someone I loved had died. Academia was an avoidance of the important things in life, which vaguely had to do with connectedness, love, meaning, and above all, simplicity. Real life was my childhood backyard—white sheets drying on a clothesline, waving in the wind on a sunny Monday morning, absorbing the scent of the lilacs growing nearby; it was watching Jake from the bedroom window as he washed his motorcycle; it was cooking *poulet sauté aux champignons* (*champion chicken*, we joked) and packing it for Jake's lunch so his fellow house painters could kid him about his *gor-may kwee-zeen*. It was in the mundane that happiness could be found. In an ordinary life.

One day I overheard our roommates, who thought I wasn't home, talking about how Jake and I were always squirreled away in the bedroom, not participating in the household, and how I was so uptight about everything—my irritation when one of them actually *used* my butcher block cutting board. I was hurt, and embarrassed about my own behavior (they were right), and then felt estranged from them.

In June, Jake and I found our own place, a tiny one-bedroom in Oakland, where I ended up lying drunk in our darkened bedroom for days on end, truly alone, willing myself to disappear inside the mattress or inside the shoes tossed in the corner, to become small, to become nothing. A grain of sand. The ultimate safety.

I succeeded quite well. Jake would come home after a day of painting houses, and I'd pour out my anxieties: What should I do now that I had dropped out of school? I had $100/month from Ian, reimbursement for my share of our car, but what if no one would hire me? Jake would say, "Don't worry about it," and it would all get stuffed back inside me, safely. For a while. I couldn't be neurotic around him. A wonderful thing, wasn't it?

I laced up my Frye boots, yellow leather—Jake had shown me the quick way to tie them, weaving both laces left to right and back again, up the long row of hooks. Part of my riding ensemble, along with my yellow helmet, for a ride north into Napa Valley to visit the wineries. Had he always been a wine connoisseur? Or only upon learning that I was an alcoholic? Swishing the wine around on our tongues and commenting on the oak, the bouquet, and then the dizzying ride home again on the twisty roads, the dip and sway as the motorcycle teased gravity on the curves.

At home, I allowed myself a bottle of wine every two days, waiting patiently until it was an acceptable time to uncork it—five o'clock, maybe four thirty. But sometimes I drank a whole bottle, lying alone in the orange light of my bedroom, reading Dostoevsky, waiting for Jake to come home. Sometimes passing out. Peeing in the wastebasket again, by mistake—or as a metaphor? Not like Jake defecating in the garden, anyway. The difference between our self-concepts.

Free from graduate school, I read the classified ads, *Help Wanted*, and ended up working for three months at the Bay Area Urban League, except I didn't understand quite how to do the job, evaluating human service programs, and so, feeling inept, I resigned and returned to a half-hearted job hunt.

With no place I wanted to go, nothing I wanted to be, I floated in space, with Jake as my lifeline. If I was nothing, I would be free—I could be anything. With no definition, all options were open to me—the ultimate freedom. Nothing to lose.

I bought a book, *Compassion and Self-Hate*, and was so embarrassed walking through the bookstore, I hid the cover so other customers couldn't see, before handing it to the store clerk. As I read it, I highlighted almost every line. But still I wasn't able to suppress my own inner critic, much less stop drinking and smoking, those habits that fed my self-hatred.

I daydreamed that maybe I could be a writer or an artist. I wrote a melodramatic short story in which the main character appeared to develop and execute a plan to murder her abusive boyfriend, drowning him in the bathtub. The murder was then revealed to be suicide, the lead character the victim in the bathtub, but the story didn't quite work, was way too dark, adding to my depression.

I drew a portrait of Jake, but the eyes weren't quite right—they looked evil. I couldn't quite capture the mystery of him. *What* mystery? His inexplicable lack of fear? His paucity of feeling (if I excepted anger)?

He lay in bed watching television while I lay next to him, whispering and sighing into his ear, "What if I can't find a job? What if—"

And Jake said, "Don't worry about it."

It was one too many times. I was enraged and grabbed a pillow and plunged it over his face to stop the words.

For once, he appeared consumed with feeling. He whipped the pillow off and yelled, "You'd better never do that again, or I might hurt you!" and he picked me up and threw me across the bed so that I almost hit the wall. But didn't.

Maybe if he'd thrown me just a touch harder, a little farther, I would have left him that night. Instead, I sat in the living room all night, huddled in a blanket, thinking about where I could go, who I could stay with, but I'd whittled my life down so I meant nothing to anyone except Jake. I sat blinded with rage and loneliness until I felt dead inside, filled with the familiar gray weight of depression, as if the abyss wasn't something I could merely fall into. It resided in me.

The night after the incident, I sat across from him at dinner, silent, while he smiled and said, "Are we friends again?"

A few months later I married him. I'd created for myself a desert island, and our relationship, whether our love was a mirage or not, was all I had protecting me from a world that seemed to have no place for me. But at what cost? I would never be reflected back from him but would simply be absorbed, light and sound into a black hole.

I moved inside Jake's dreams because I had none of my own. I encouraged him to start the health food store he longed to own and manage. Researched how to do it. Wrote the Small

Business Administration. Taught myself bookkeeping and accounting. Developed a business plan, with Jake's narrative and my financial statements showing it would work.

I was sitting at the kitchen table, tackling some paperwork required for our business, when Jake came home from work. I said, "I have to identify the type of business we're starting."

"Just write 'sole proprietor.'" He was covered in paint dust, probably toxic, from grinding the exterior of someone's house, and sat down to remove his work boots. He looked up when I was silent. "What is it?"

"I assumed we'd be partners. After all, we're married."

"But it's my expertise. And my money." He had managed a health food store in San Francisco.

"But what about all the work I've put into the start-up? That should count for something."

"I could have done that myself. I didn't ask you to do that."

"Yeah, sure, like you would have learned bookkeeping and accounting, and—"

"I appreciate what you did, but it's not brain science."

"Technically, if we're married, I think everything is jointly owned."

"Maybe in California."

"Oh, go fuck yourself. You're such an asshole."

We ate dinner in silence.

Then he sighed. "Okay, we can be partners, I guess."

"We supposedly *are* partners."

"In the sense that we're married."

"So I'll say fifty/fifty on the forms. We have to specify the percentage of ownership."

He laughed. "I was thinking more like ninety/ten."

"After I've done eighty percent of the work so far? No way—you can just go to Boston on your own then."

"But what if we got divorced? You could wipe me out if it was fifty/fifty."

"Right now I'd be happy to divorce you."

"Eighty/twenty then."

As much as I wanted to believe that as married partners we co-owned everything and were equals, I didn't feel that way. I hadn't saved any money and felt less-than because I couldn't contribute as much. It was *his* savings we were investing, and I could partly see his logic. I capitulated. But still it galled me that he so underestimated my value to the partnership. Anyway, we were married, so we'd either jointly rake in the dough or go bankrupt.

We decided to move to Boston, near Jake's family, where there would be less competition than there was in the San Francisco area. A new beginning. Giving up everything for a fresh start. Again.

CHAPTER 7:

THE MOTHER HOOD

How easy it was for a life to go astray. How easy it was to get into my 1965 VW Bug with Jake and ride into the unknown.

On our way to Massachusetts, we stayed one night with Mom and Peter, who'd recently moved back from California to Sylvan Grove, Wisconsin. The highlight was Mom pulling me aside to complain about Jake's bad table manners, serving himself before everyone even sat down.

It was thirty-five below zero when we left the next morning. By the time Jake had pushed the Bug to a sluggish start, his mustache had turned white with icicles. The accelerator felt like a worn-out sponge, stiff with cold under my foot. Perhaps it had been an omen. Perhaps we should've simply turned around, but a blizzard held us captive—we couldn't even exit the highway because of the drifts. The hood of the Bug, a dingy white, was barely distinguishable from the mounds of snow flowing away from us in all directions, the flakes so thick that it felt like driving through the interior of a feather mattress. Ohio was a shroud of white punctuated only by the carcasses of semis tipped into roadside ditches, which at least allowed me to identify the road so I could move along it by connecting the dots, truck to truck.

For a while, our life in Boston was electric with activity, the frenzy of finding a store location, getting a business loan, negotiating a mall lease, finding an apartment in Watertown, purchasing fixtures, equipment, and inventory (natural foods, herbal and vitamin supplements, including our own label), and opening the store despite the last-minute switch of venue to a larger, more expensive space than we wanted, orchestrated by the mall owners. Jake and I were both engrossed, working very long hours, but functioning smoothly as a team. And almost immediately I'd become pregnant, and within the year my life had settled into a monotone, like the white of the blizzard, opaque, thick, hidden.

I was stunned by my own fertility. I'd taken foolish risks all those years ago, somehow assuming my body wasn't capable of pregnancy, partly because I hadn't *planned* it. How lucky I'd been that first year at UW–Madison, when I'd lost my virginity in the front seat of a Mustang while in a drunken stupor, lying across the emergency brake, William smiling and saying he'd marry me if I got pregnant, and my mild retort, "*That* won't be necessary." Sneaking into the boys' dorm with Richard, and his discovery that *Oops, the rubber broke.*

And then, accompanying my friend Ginny to the office of a ninety-year-old doctor, who examined both of us and told Ginny, "Someone sure knocked you up good," before turning to me and chuckling, "But you don't ever have to worry about a bun in your oven, because you have an underdeveloped uterus. Unless maybe you take some of those new-fangled fertility pills."

Just as I'd always thought—I wasn't a real woman. I'd been a late developer, last to need a bra, last to menstruate, and now I'd been told I couldn't have kids. Real women had to travel to a secret address, where they applied a special knock to a plain wooden door and gave the password; where they lay on a kitchen table, legs flung apart, their mistakes scraped clean out of them, the bloody mass with tiny, animal features shown to them, then flushed. Sworn to secrecy and then ushered to the door, wobbling hours later into the dorm, pale with loss.

Within days of the baby's conception, my tender, swollen breasts convinced me I was pregnant. I'd recently visited my gynecologist after one of my regular checks revealed that my IUD was no longer positioned properly, but instead was lodged in my cervix. When he removed it, he said he was surprised I wasn't pregnant. Days later I realized I was.

Jake just laughed. "You're not pregnant—you're just imagining things. It's not an opportune time anyway."

"I *am* pregnant. I know I am." I was certain, despite my supposed infertility and even though I'd discovered tiny drops of blood. My breasts told me so.

"We can talk about it if and when it becomes reality."

When a blood test proved me right, I rejoiced—I was joining the ranks of womanhood with my newfound normality—I could have a child! Jake wanted to consider abortion, but while I was pro-choice, I found I couldn't seriously consider it. Maybe my pregnancy was a fluke, a miracle, and God/fate had meant for this particular child to be born, had displaced my IUD. Maybe I'd been given this one chance and there would never be another. Or maybe I was solely responsible—once I thought I might be pregnant, I wanted a baby so much that I thought maybe I had willed the blood away, willed this new life into existence. The store be damned, I would have this baby.

I carefully drove back and forth to the store, avoiding potholes, avoiding the fumes of trucks and buses, willing my uterus to hold the embryo in place, to grow large beyond its predicted capacity. After seeing the doctor, I went immediately to the bookstore and bought Dr. Spock's *Baby and Child Care*, as well as *The First Nine Months of Life*, *The Nursing Mother*, *The Mother Person*, *The Mother Knot*, and *How to Parent*, to add to my worn-in copy of *Our Bodies, Ourselves*, and then settled myself in an easy chair and prepared to cloak myself under the mother hood for the next five to twenty years.

Pregnancy was a grand thing. Wondrous, to feel another body inside me, to imagine a miniature person becoming whole in there. I donned my green velvet string bikini so Jake could take a belly photo in our dining room, and for another, I stood (fully dressed) with my arms raised to the sky on a rock overlooking the Charles River—*See me, I am woman.* After all. While business associates at the store just thought I was letting myself go.

Like other babies, my baby—a girl I was told by an acupuncturist visiting the store who swung a key chain above my belly—would be born a *tabula rasa*, and she would be shaped by my love and attention to become a fully realized person, all that she could be. I was shocked when Jessica emerged after seven hours of my blowing and panting like a cornetist playing an eternal vivace, while staring at a Sierra Club photo of a moon shining through a dark forest. Seven hours of agony, without drugs ("natural" childbirth, only the best for my baby), assured me my insides were being ripped apart by the silver tools of a crazed car mechanic. I asked, "Why doesn't she have a chin? She looks like Grandpa Gerald." Jessie, two weeks late and covered with what looked like white phlegm, was wrinkled like an old man, but with a shock of dark hair and Jake's black eyes.

Her chin popped out a few days later, and I quickly learned that even infants had minds of their own. This I called *the temperament theory*—they were *born* with a disposition and genetics had to be given their due after all. Jessie rarely slept, and she nursed almost nonstop for the next eighteen months, so that my fondest desires were to never be touched again and to sleep for eight full hours.

I hadn't quite realized the commitment I was making. The shock to our lifestyle was so profound that the only explanation had to be the existence of a universal conspiracy to prevent potential parents from knowing what parenthood really meant. After Jessie was born, I stopped brushing my teeth because I didn't have time. I learned to eat peas with a fork held in my left hand while Jessie clung to my right breast; learned not to roll onto her as she lay propped between Jake and me, attached to me even in sleep; learned to pack whenever I had to step outside the front door: diapers, wipes, juice bottle, snacks, toys, change of clothes. Getting into the car, getting out of the car—a major ordeal. Strapping the baby in, unstrapping the baby, then loading her into a Snugli, a baby carriage, a stroller, or over my hip. Learning which places I could go with a baby (the library, the mall, an outdoor movie) and which places I couldn't (good restaurants, theaters). Because I could never be sure how long I'd have before my sweet baby metamorphosed into a voracious animal, screaming with need.

I turned off my radio for years, because the baby was sleeping, or *just in case* Jessie (and two years later, Brandon) might sleep, so that I could also sleep, finally. It occurred to me that mothers . . . couldn't even finish a thought . . . never mind read a full sentence . . . without interruption. Not only was I denied my dreams by the disruption of REM sleep (and wasn't that supposed to lead to emotional problems?), I was denied my opportunity to think. Maybe that was why mothers were often considered nonentities—their minds had dissolved into thought-free reverie when at last they'd exhausted their attempts to remain thinking human beings with a right to a life of their own.

There was no greater responsibility than having kids. Half of my exhaustion was from the constant vigilance I had to maintain. Just to keep the baby alive. Was the baby breathing? Would she tear the button nose off the stuffed dachshund, try to eat it, and choke to death? Would she become ensnared in the blankets and smother? Would she choke on bagel crumbs? When she became mobile, crawling—the danger of the bare electric outlet, of the blades of the fan, of television wires that could be chewed, of hot radiators, of kitchen knives within reach, of tasty cleanser and bleach, of objects pulled off tables and falling on the tender *O* of her head—the fontanel, that filmy curtain over the brain, that seemed a doorway to potential death. Because, after all, horrible things could happen if you turned your back. If I'd been watching, maybe my brother wouldn't have killed himself. It couldn't happen twice to me, it just couldn't. I couldn't live with it twice. Once was an accident maybe, this turning away at a crucial moment, but twice was a plan. Or at least negligence. And which moment was crucial? Those were the downsides of parenthood.

The upside was the miracle of life, created by me, unfolding in front of me, so that I could almost believe in God. When I really thought about it, just the physical aspects of conception, development, and birth, the sperm with its microscopic plans plunging into an egg that had other plans, the merging into one living cell, floating down a red river and attaching itself to the uterine wall in just the right place, the millionfold division of cells into a predestined shape, the ultimate birth of consciousness, a human being emerging from the inside of another human being, it was truly astounding. The miles of capillaries, an intricate transportation system feeding millions of cells; the mystery of eyesight, an eyeball—a spherical ball of tissue and fluid that can communicate what's out there; the heart, a perpetual motion machine for perhaps a hundred years—how could it have all happened by chance?

Motherhood was heaven and hell, both. I told my childless friends in letters that the children had saved my life. Suicide was no longer an option; I could never ever abandon my children. I wanted them to feel totally loved, to learn everything they needed to become all they could be, to have everything I could give them, to be safe from harm.

For Jessie, I made my own baby food, grinding organic grains into cereal and cooking, pureeing, and freezing organic meats into ice cubes so no chemicals would pass her lips. I sank into bitter self-condemnation that my smoke still polluted Jessie's air, that I couldn't quite give up my nightly wine that must surely seep into my breast milk, although still Jessie barely slept.

I made her a mobile of flying birds to hang above her crib, a quilt, and curtains for her room; hung posters of animals and flowers; bought educational toys, puzzles, and plastic books for her to look at and chew and finger paints so she could express herself; surrounded her with furry stuffed animals and toys that tinkled, sang, and made animal noises so her room became a jumble of color, sound, pattern, and texture.

I nursed first Jessie and then Brandon to sleep each night, and later Jake or I sat with them and told them stories by the light of their Snoopy night-light until they fell asleep, so they wouldn't have to be alone with their fears, so they wouldn't huddle as I did as a child, head covered, only my nose exposed to the dark air, sure that someone would come stab me in the night. Picked them up whenever they cried, thinking that if I met their dependency needs now, they'd grow into independent people. That if I was sensitive to their emotional needs, they might grow up normal and not lose their minds and kill themselves. Potential genetic fate hung over their lives like a guillotine ready to fall, if I wasn't very, very careful.

The disorder of children, their free-wheeling desire to get into everything, to throw, drop, break things, made me want to scream. Scraping congealed cereal and cottage cheese from the cracks in the wooden high chair, from the floor, from the nearby table, I imagined a self-contained unit with an overhead shower that would simply wash the mess away. I took a photo of Jessie standing on a pile of books she'd cleared from the bookshelves, and later mourned the torn covers and apple juice stains but didn't want to discourage her curiosity, her exploration of her environment, so essential to her growth as a child.

I became overwhelmed with a sense of futility, a wave of depression, upon entering the children's room and seeing every single toy scraped off the shelves into a sea of wood and plastic that covered the floor, hundreds, maybe thousands of tiny toys that I would then put away, knowing they would only be flung around the room the next day.

Once, when Jessie was a baby and woke me up for the fifth time in one night, I barely resisted my fantasy of throwing her back into the crib and, with a pillow (that pillow again), stifling those cries that seemed to say, *You have to gimme more, more, more*, when I felt I had nothing left to give. I'd already given my whole life.

But it was the fear of what might happen to the children that kept me at home, doing the store bookkeeping and accounting late at night, not adherence to what I considered repugnant traditional values.

I hadn't counted on the never-ending poverty, on the bare survival lifestyle. When we opened the store, Jake and I pictured ourselves either rolling in profit or going bankrupt, not the in-between state of just surviving. We couldn't afford to go to movies or restaurants or plays or museums. I owned one pair of jeans, two pairs of footwear—sandals for summer, boots for winter—two tops for summer, a couple of old sweaters for winter, and two old pairs of dress slacks.

Photos in summer always showed me wearing a spaghetti-strap burgundy camisole, jeans, and sandals, my long straight hair tied back into a long ponytail. When we had to go to Jake's cousin's wedding, I wore a maternity blouse, the unnecessary fabric draped loosely over the belt.

I resisted eating certain foods, fruit, snacks, because I thought of them as being *for the kids*. I had trouble justifying buying anything for myself and spent money only on cigarettes (forty-seven cents a pack) and wine, those things I couldn't live without.

I thought about looking for a job, but I was nursing, and first Jessie, then Brandon, wouldn't take a bottle, and besides, there was the accounting to do, the cost of childcare, and the promise of screaming terror if I left the kids with someone else. I'd seen it already when Jake and I left the kids with their nana, Teri, Jake's mother. I decided I just couldn't leave them—that I would be abandoning them. I would never, never, be like my own mother. A little hard to reconcile with my feminist self, the charter subscriber to *Ms.* magazine, the former Berkeley consciousness-raising group member, the author of a professional journal article on sex stereotypes and role standards (I had demanded, and was granted, first authorship), someone who had refused to let a man open a door for her just a few years before, but I rationalized this by deciding it was okay for other women to choose to return to work, but as for me, why, it was my *choice* to stay at home.

I dimly recalled a time when I was irritated by women who argued about the validity of the role of stay-at-home mother and wife—why would anyone want to do that, to become a boring drudge? But there I was, a boring drudge myself, wrapped in a cloak of invisibility as I strolled my baby down the street—I was a role, not a person, not someone you'd notice. The upside was the streets seemed safer—no one (I thought then) would attack a mother with a child. I was protected by my children. When I met people who asked what I did for a living, they immediately lost interest, so I was saved from my own shyness, dismissed from the expectation of clever conversation.

One Thanksgiving, at Jake's parents' house, the men clustered in the living room and discussed real estate and sports, as was usual, while the women prepared dinner in the kitchen and talked about kids, redecorating. My brother- and sister-in-law had arrived without the expected pumpkin pie—she'd thrown it at her husband. Although peeved we wouldn't have pie, I admired her audacity, and it spurred me on. I was annoyed with the stereotypical division of labor vs. "non-labor," so at first I tried just sitting with the men, resisting the urge to help, although I thought everyone should. But bored and excluded, I caved and joined the kitchen crew.

After dinner, as the men began to stand, I said, "Why don't you men do the dishes? We did all the cooking." Which earned a wide-eyed silence from both men and women that implied I must be joking. But the moment quickly dissolved—into a pretense that I hadn't actually said anything at all, as conversation resumed. I felt I'd been painted into a still life, every figure immutably stationed in its *appropriate* place. As if we were all only caricatures, outlines of people.

This was the *ordinary life*, the one in which I couldn't be *neurotic* because Jake wouldn't look too deeply into me, that had attracted me to him in the first place. As often seemed to happen, that first alluring quality had morphed into what now felt like a deal-breaker.

Even the friendships we made (Donna, Bea, Sara, and their husbands) were via having a baby—other parents-to-be in our natural childbirth class—friends that were not chosen but thrown together by virtue of our biological rhythms. There were family get-togethers, with husbands, wives, and babies, and although I felt a little of that anti-family tug, a little death of self in the context of the traditional roles we were ambitiously trying to don like new costumes, I enjoyed the camaraderie. But mostly we arranged mother-baby afternoons together, outings to Nursing Mothers Council meetings, lunches at each other's houses, babies laid out on blankets on living room floors for indoor picnic lunches, the mothers surrounded by toys and diaper bags, immersed in conversations about rashes and sleeping habits and which baby had learned to roll over first, and I contributed too, but inside was asking myself: *What am I doing here? Do I still exist?*

I watched as other mothers became breastfeeding counselors or birth attendants, and tried to imagine myself making the birth process or nursing the center of my life, but couldn't. I was different, already an outsider—no one had spotted me as a natural talent, a starlet-to-be sitting at the Schwab's drugstore counter awaiting my role in the great mother/baby show. Others had been called, recruited, but not me. Maybe I failed in some way to exude the proper motherliness.

The weight of twenty-four-hour alertness and attention to the needs of my kids became almost more than I could bear.

Jake was gone from morning until late at night, working mall hours, Monday through Saturday. I sometimes raged at him when he went motorcycle riding on Sundays with his brothers, but he would say things like, "I deserve my morning off. I'm working hard to support my family." And I'd yell back, "You don't think caring for two kids is work?" And he'd say, "It doesn't seem so tough to me, hanging around the house and visiting with your friends."

The playgroups metamorphosed into two-hour babysitting exchanges. I lived for my two hours of freedom every other week, time just for myself, but after handing over my kids and walking out the door of Donna's or Sara's or Bea's house, praying I could make it out of hearing distance without the cries of my children tugging at my heart, I felt a dread—the clock was already ticking and I had to use this time in a meaningful way—and then futility. What could I accomplish in two hours that would be a meaningful use of my time? Once I subtracted travel time, there was little time left, and my only friends were busy—taking care of my children and theirs. Usually I decided to run errands, so much simpler, quicker, when I didn't have to drag the kids and their equipment along. Sometimes I went home and lay on my bed staring out the window wondering, *Is this all there is?*

The summer after Brandon turned one, Jake and I finally decided to sell the store. The break-even point kept climbing, largely due to a variable interest rate that soared from 6 percent to 22 percent while sales declined—we weren't bringing in enough money to keep up the inventory, so we lost customers.

Increasingly, I drank. I watched the clock until four or five, poured my first glass of burgundy into a brandy snifter, then felt the relief as the wine slid down my throat and removed me a few inches from the life I'd made. When Jake finally came home and could be the responsible parent, I could drink freely, though I tried to be discreet about my refills, until I crashed onto our bed, dizzy and lost somewhere else, inside a dream of my life, inside my mind.

Sometimes Jake would open the closed bedroom door, find me lying on the cold, wooden floor, and pull me up and lay me on the bed without ever saying a word. Maybe he simply thought my drinking was none of his business. Maybe he thought of me as another bottle of vitamins fallen from the shelf, or maybe he didn't think of me at all. And it was my responsibility, my shame. But I couldn't stop. Watched the clock until it was time, waiting for my little bit of freedom.

While pregnant with Jessie, I'd worried about my drinking and smoking and cut down on both as much as I could but was afraid the damage had already been done—I was drinking heavily before I discovered I was pregnant. I'd even gone through Smokenders, and earned the unique status of being the only participant still attending who smoked right to the end, at which point one of the leaders looked at my belly and warned that she'd suffered a stillbirth because of her own smoking, and did I want that to happen? I'd simply walked out, trying to appear untouched, and only cried as I was driving home in the car. I just couldn't seem to quit my bad habits.

Right before my pregnancy with Brandon, I successfully quit drinking, wanting to avoid the anguish, the fantasies of deformed children. Later, when we dared to dream of buying a house, a broken-down cottage on a lake in need of significant repair, but then realized we couldn't afford it even if his parents cosigned the loan, Jake brought home a bottle of brandy for himself, and I decided I'd join him just that once. During the next two years, I socked away bottle after bottle of wine or sometimes brandy. But discreetly. Even my friends didn't know.

As our life seemed to fall apart, the failing store, our inability to afford a house, being stuck at home with two toddlers, I thought about leaving Jake, but I had trouble justifying it, because he wasn't *obviously* a bad person—people were forever calling him a nice guy. But we had little in common other than our sexual compatibility, and the electricity had gradually faded as my unspoken grievances mounted. It was more a matter of what was missing. Omissions.

Jake and I sat in an ice cream parlor in silence. He curved his mouth into a half smile and looked at me from the corner of his eyes, with a knowing look that didn't refer to anything said or lead to conversation. It was the thing in and of itself, a still life of Jake making a certain face to give the illusion of meaning. I looked into his eyes, eyes like holes into a vacuum that could suck me right in, and then I grasped the table edge, foolishly, and tore my gaze away, as if my whole body might fly over the table and be pulled inside that darkness, those empty brown eyes sitting in such a handsome, swarthy face.

I detested Jake for little things. For walking ahead of me on the street. For turning off lights in rooms where I sat. For silencing the radio, shutting off the music that connected me like an umbilical cord to the world outside my home, the songs that reminded me that there was such a thing as love, maybe. For dropping his motorcycle boots from a height of two feet to the bedroom floor and bouncing onto our bed, shaking me out of my dreams. For his truisms. For saying, *What's on the menu? What's new on the home front?* Over and over again. For saying words twice, as if it meant he was saying more: *Good, good*, when I said I was okay, when okay didn't mean good at all. For things he did *not* do: leaving the porch light on for me; asking me what I thought, what I felt; laughing at my humor. Because he couldn't sing, and for some reason I believed that all good men could sing.

I hated him for calling me his rubber raft, causing the plug to pop right out of my sexual fantasies. For walking down the street and looking at his own lanky reflection in the dark windows, stroking his villainous mustache. I looked at Jake, ready to smile at him, expecting him to look back at me, but instead found him staring at himself. For saying *I* instead of *we*. For saying *he'd* been on vacation, *he* had bills to pay, *he'd* written the business plan. History apparently had been rewritten: I hadn't been in New Hampshire after all, hadn't labored over the family budget or paid the bills, hadn't slaved over the plan. I was dead after all, but no one had told me, so I'd just hung around, a ghost mistaken about my own identity.

I just didn't seem able to affect him, couldn't get him to see me, and maybe that arose from a deficit in me—a lack of substance or character. Maybe a steady drip of being treated like I was nothing created a deep hole of actual nothingness—a true emptiness. I was a mist with a name—*Dear*, *Babe*, sometimes *Bitch*. When it was *Bitch*, at least I felt I existed. But I probably expected too much of him, perfection. Maybe I didn't love him well enough, didn't try hard enough, but he often *said* he loved me, and then I'd say, "Love isn't just a feeling. It's an act."

I thought of leaving him but couldn't see how. I wondered whether I'd feel different about him if I quit smoking. Maybe then I'd feel different about myself, be rid of my self-loathing for smoking, which Jake so often reminded me was polluting the kids' and his air. I avoided kissing him anymore, because he hated the taste. I was thin, maybe gaunt, and I joked that I only allowed myself to abuse non-nutritional substances—calorie-free coffee, the hazy ether of smoke, vitamin-free alcohol, as if the goal were to avoid supplying any sustenance at all, anything that would detract from the refrigerator and add to my frame. As if the goal were to fade from visibility altogether. If I could give up smoking, alcohol would be the only need I had left, the only incursion I made on the family budget. I was approaching the perfection of my long-sought state of nothingness.

And now Jake was bugging me to go see a hypnotist, someone he'd known years ago.

PART III:

KNOW ME, 1981–1982

CHAPTER 8:

STOLEN CARS AND FROZEN SUPERHEROES

Sam hadn't been my therapist at first. Just an acquaintance of Jake's from college days who had come into the store with his wife, Joy. According to Jake, Sam had offered to hypnotize me, free of charge, to help me quit smoking. Jake thought we might all become friends.

When I arrived at Sam's house for my appointment, I thought, *This place should be mine.* His house was the upscale mirror image of our downscale, peeling-paint house, brown-shingled like ours, but a single-family. I rang the bell and entered, as the sign told me, but worried whether the instruction applied at such an ungodly hour, 7:00 a.m.

I coughed a little so Sam would know I was in the foyer and checked my appearance in a mirror framed by stained glass flowers, with a lone flower emerging into the center of the mirror itself—a suggestion to see the "flower" within? I could hear footsteps above and a radio playing classical music.

I'd imagined Sam would be tall and dark—he had such a deep voice over the phone—but when he descended the stairs, saying hello as if he was very glad to see me, I felt a touch of disappointment. He was of average height with a stocky build, maybe carrying an extra pound or two, with auburn hair and a beard that I thought was a little much—Freud, etc. That was when I realized I'd wanted him to be attractive. Already he seemed intrigued with me, the way he'd spoken on the phone with exclamation marks—*Ambivalent!*—when I said I was ambivalent about quitting smoking.

When he asked me if I wanted coffee, I followed him right into his kitchen, sat at the kitchen table, and watched him grind the coffee beans. Later, I thought maybe it had been a faux pas on my part.

Coffee in hand, I followed him upstairs as he placed each foot softly on each step—gracefully or self-consciously, I wasn't sure which. Much later, I thought *reverently*, as if each footstep would ripple through the world, as if one must be very, very careful, very, very gentle, because every motion was a holy act.

At the top, he turned left into a sunlit room, which contained hanging plants, a bookcase, artwork on white walls, two plush armchairs to my left, separated from what I assumed was his chair by a corner table with a lamp, clock, tissues—and an ashtray, to my relief. I sat in the chair closest to his.

That first visit in September, significant on my calendar because it was the autumnal equinox, we chatted. He was a clinical psychologist, having earned his doctorate a few years before, and after I told him I'd gone to grad school in psychology at Berkeley, only in personality research, we compared notes.

Sam said, "I found the writing difficult. Didn't you?"

"Not at all. It was the orals that worried me."

He nodded. "That can be a difficult hurdle. Are you originally from California?"

"No, I just went to school there, UCLA, then Berkeley. I'm from a tiny town, Houston, in Wisconsin, where my father was a turkey farmer."

"I'm from turkey country too. In Vermont. And how did you end up in Massachusetts?"

"Jake and I met in Berkeley, and then when I dropped out, we decided to move here to open the store. Less competition, we thought. And his family's here."

We both smoked, I my Merits, he his pipe. I thought it was a bit hypocritical of him.

"What does smoking mean to you?" he asked.

I riffed, "It's my fuel, my comfort, my lifelong companion, visible evidence that I exist, a protective barrier, a clue that something is wrong, a spitting at the world—engaging in what is now a socially undesirable habit, my way of living on the edge, just between life and death, teasing death."

"You've put some thought into this." He smiled.

"And of course there's the oral fixation, as Freud would say."

"Are you a fan of his work?"

"I used to pooh-pooh it, like a lot of people, as outdated and so on, but I learned to appreciate some of his ideas when I was a teaching assistant for a class focused on his original writings."

"I'm impressed. His work can be difficult to grasp. I agree he contributed important ideas to the field."

"About smoking. Underneath all those reasons to smoke, the truth is I'm terribly addicted. I'm not sure what hypnosis can do about that."

"You might find it a useful tool to assist in addressing the addiction."

I was doubtful, but what did I have to lose.

At the second visit, Sam tape-recorded his attempt to hypnotize me. I wasn't sure it worked—I was too self-conscious about having my eyes closed, thinking he might be looking me over. He included stop-smoking suggestions and gave me the tape to take home.

I protested, "How can I use it with the kids around all the time?"

He suggested, "Maybe you can include them in some way in the process."

He obviously didn't have kids.

I tried the tape a couple of times that week, holing up in the bedroom, lying in the darkness, listening to his deep voice, while Jake watched the kids in the living room. It felt like sleeping with another man in front of Jake. When Sam's voice talked me through the relaxation of my body, from toes to head, I noticed a halting in his voice in one or two places, as if I'd been right—he *had* been studying my body. I pictured him, and no, he wasn't conventionally handsome, but he looked at me and seemed to *see* me, listened to me intently and seemed to *hear* me, so already I felt a little naked in his gaze, somehow revealed. His demeanor, his interest, feigned or not, surprised me.

It was a half-hearted attempt at best, trying to quit smoking to appease Jake and to relieve my own guilt. I felt far more shame about the alcohol. I'd get up for those early morning sessions with Sam and rub a rough washcloth over my lips, trying to abrade the cells coated with wine and nicotine stains, and stick some gum in my mouth to mask the alcoholic fumes that oozed from my body. Funny I didn't spontaneously combust when I lit my first cigarette of the day.

After a couple of meetings, I said I didn't want to use the tape during the session—I just couldn't get into it. He said he thought there might be some other issues I wanted to work on, that I seemed so sad.

"Yes. I'm an alcoholic. And I hate my life." I sighed. "But paying would be a problem."

"I'm sure we can work something out."

"And there's something else bothering me, a lump in my throat, *globus hystericus*—one of my Berkeley friends said Freud had called it that—and only drinking gives me any relief. Such a weird symptom."

"It's not so weird." And then he mumbled, "I myself have a phobia of cloth dolls."

"Cloth dolls?"

He nodded, looking little-boyishly vulnerable, a bit embarrassed. "I only meant that many people have unusual symptomatology. It's not so rare."

"I suppose my lump means there's something I need to say." I smiled.

Sam suggested we try a less directed hypnosis to see what might surface, and then led me through the usual steps, instructing me to tighten and then release each set of muscles from my toes to my head, and then asking how relaxed I was on a scale of one to ten.

"I . . . I feel unable to open my mouth," I said through barely parted lips.

"You'll be able to speak, and when an image or sensation enters your awareness, you'll describe it."

How could he know that? He seemed so sure. I sat silently lost in space, in time. My eyes still closed, I said, "There . . . is . . . a . . . small . . . light." Above Sam's chair, to my left.

I heard him move forward in his chair. "Where is it? Can you show me?"

I lifted my arm. "I . . . I . . . can't reach it." I withdrew my hand.

"What would you like to do with the light?"

"I want it closer."

"Can you invite it to come to you?"

I concentrated. The light floated down and sat in my cupped hands. "It's such a tiny light. It's white. A tiny white light." My eyes filled with tears.

"What will you do with it?"

"I'm supposed to absorb it, through here." I placed my right hand over my heart/stomach area. "But I can't. It has nothing to do with me."

"Nothing to do with you?"

Tears rolled down my cheeks. "I can only hold it in my hand. And caress it."

"What does the light mean to you?"

I thought for a moment, squeezing back the tears. "It is . . . life. A kind of vitality. A pure energy." *Love maybe?*

"Are you aware of anything else about this little light?"

I smiled. "I have an impulse to eat it."

"Why don't you?"

"It's not the right way. It can only be absorbed. A kind of osmosis."

"What will you do with the light then?"

"It seems to be fading a little. I want to set it free." I lifted it with my hand and let it float off to my right.

When I was awake again, I said I thought the whole thing was weird, that I felt silly. But Sam called it *a very powerful experience.*

And it wasn't over. On the way home, I strained at the wheel, hunched over it, fighting a persistent impulse to drive head-on into oncoming cars. Maybe the little light was the lump set free. But maybe I needed it right where it had been, in my throat—for protection.

Jake eyed me from the kitchen table when I arrived home. "How was your meeting with Sam?"

"Fine." I shouldn't have to tell him everything that went on there.

"I see you're still smoking." He smiled.

Yeah, as if I should have kicked the habit after only two sessions. I ignored him.

In our next session, Sam asked about my drinking. I said I'd started drinking in my first year of college, had been a "good girl" until then, but had binged along with everyone else when I finally escaped the small-town mores and gossip-mongering that mostly kept people in line or at least encouraged secrecy.

"But drinking didn't become a problem until later. I had a brother, a year younger than me, who committed suicide. Shot himself in the head with a rifle. It marked the 'before and after' in my life. Oh, and I have a sister, too, Mandy, who's five and a half years younger than me."

"That must have been very tough for you and your family."

"Right at the top of my list of bad things that have happened to me. He'd been diagnosed with paranoid schizophrenia a couple of years before and was worried he'd never get his mind back, so he took what I guess he thought was his only way out."

"And your drinking escalated then?"

"Not exactly. I didn't even have time to think about Brian. Right after his funeral, Ian, my first husband, and I moved to Berkeley for grad school, and then I was inundated with coursework and prepping to teach discussion sections."

"You were a TA your first year?"

I nodded. "Without any training. I was terrified and worked constantly to be prepared for those sessions, never mind my own classes. I'd drink a dozen cups of coffee and get so jittery I had to drink a ton of wine to calm down."

I sighed. "I know drinking is just another form of escape, to forget my own misery, my inability to wrest control of my life. Not unlike escaping my first marriage, grad school, California. When I was talking to one of my advisors about leaving grad school, I referred to it as a form of escape, a failure of fortitude or something, and he said, 'Sometimes escape works.'"

"He gave you permission . . ."

"Yes. I felt so relieved. He made walking away seem like a valid option, not a failure on my part. The problem was, I didn't know what to escape *to*."

I looked out his window and let my mind wander.

"What are you thinking right now?"

"When I was in high school, the principal and guidance counselor called me to the office specifically to tell me, 'We think you can become whatever you want to be.' In a moment of youthful arrogance, I thought that much was already obvious. But what did I want? I didn't know then and I guess I still don't."

Ever since high school, I'd repeatedly tossed my life into the wind to see where I'd land. Fifteen years later, there I sat, complaining to Sam, my life as stagnant as the old Houston pond. Drinking, my only relief from what felt like multiple forms of failure.

"Tell me a little about your first marriage." I gave him an abbreviated version; we were good friends, but missing chemistry, and I felt too much like his mother or sister.

"And how is it different with Jake?"

"The chemistry is, or was, there, but I'm not sure anymore if there's anything else."

Thanksgiving morning 1981. I awoke feeling alien to this life, as if I were merely an actress who'd been plunked down into a very convincing setting. Although I knew my lines, they weren't my own words. I felt as though I'd been transported from another life but given the necessary historical information to recognize the children, their names, the titles of books on my bookshelves, and the recipe for green beans almondine I needed for my contribution to dinner at my mother-in-law's house.

All was unreal to me. How could it be that I was here? I thought I was going crazy—the word "crazy" seemed less onerous than "mentally ill," a little lighter, as if it might be a fun way to be. I'd always been afraid that I might, just like Brian. Or maybe I'd drunk the critical drop of alcohol—the one that pushed me over some threshold, damaged one too many brain cells so the ruin had now reached an observable level.

I hadn't drunk much the night before, so it couldn't be a hangover, but instead must be a permanent pickling of my brain, and I thought, *My mind is all I could ever count on.* It was my intelligence that showered me with goodies when nothing else seemed to work. Now maybe my mind was gone forever too. Exactly what Brian must have felt once he was lucid enough to assess the condition of his mind.

When I stopped drinking for good that day, babying myself with Fresca, snacks, and stolen naps, it was not a courageous act. I simply didn't dare to drink another drop. What I was most afraid of losing, not counting my kids, might already be lost. I often quoted Martin Heidegger to myself: "The dreadful has already happened." Brian's suicide. But there appeared to be other losses in store.

When I told Sam I'd quit drinking, he was excited about what he considered a breakthrough, while I felt my life had merely slid a few inches further down the tunnel to the abyss. Brain damage wasn't something I could feel excited about. When he wanted Jake to join our next session, because *repercussions would be felt in the family*, I simply felt resentful—couldn't I ever have anything all to myself? And cynical—who knew how long this would last? I'd quit before, a couple of times.

At the meeting, Sam asked Jake if I'd told him I wanted to focus on some other issues besides smoking, and I was embarrassed. I hadn't said a word to Jake, afraid he'd say no—the money. But Jake said it was okay as long as it didn't go on too long—therapy was okay for a while, but then he thought people should get on with their lives. I thought, *What life?*

When we left, Jake patted Sam on the back. Making like friends, I thought. So gauche.

I started to dream the nights before my sessions, and I joked with Sam, "As if I wanted to bring you a present." I huddled down in the deep plush chair and told him my dreams, including one I'd had a few months before starting therapy.

> *I'm kneeling with Brandon before the open refrigerator, while Jessie and a friend stand in the doorway. Suddenly, items from the fridge are flying across the room. The children scream. I realize I'm causing the objects to fly around and quickly shut the refrigerator door. The food falls to the floor. I see Brandon's and my reflection in the metal of the door. A deep voice comes from my mouth, a male voice, saying, "Come home from my body, Mama, so I can't eat you anymore." Then I scream.*

I told Sam I'd recorded the dream in my journal because it was so weird.

When he prodded a little, I said, "I think it was Brian's voice. It might have been him and me kneeling before the refrigerator, which might symbolize our cold mother. She was always wearing sweaters, standing in front of the heat register, signing 'From Mother' on Christmas gifts. Maybe he was addressing her? Or maybe it was Brian telling me to let go of him, of his suicide."

"Rich dreams," Sam said. "You're a very complex woman."

I told him what it was like in our childhood kitchen, the scene of many crimes: my father's silence, my mother's interrogations of him, *Why didn't he talk to her, why hadn't he told her the news she'd had to pick up elsewhere*, my father's grunts in response; both my parents ranting repeatedly at Brian to get a haircut, my mother debasing him, telling him he'd never amount to anything.

"Your mother could be difficult?" Sam asked.

"Neither of my husbands could stand to be around her for long. She constantly nitpicks or harangues—my dad, Brian, and I were all targets, Mandy not so much, and now my mother has Peter to nag. She doesn't seem aware of what she's doing."

"What was it like for you?"

I thought for a moment. "Do you think first memories are significant?"

He nodded.

"I was three, running wildly around the dining room table, my brother chasing me, while my mother practiced the piano for church—she was the pianist. I turned to see how close Brian was and, in my distraction, smashed my head into a doorframe. Blood spurted all over my Sunday clothes. My mother grabbed a washcloth, plastered it to my head, and then collapsed on the floor with Brian and me, and we all wailed together.

"But she was probably crying and complaining about my getting blood all over my Sunday dress, about how she'd have to find someone to play the piano for her, and why did things like this always happen to her? Everything was always about her, not me. She didn't even bother to take me to the doctor for stitches.

"See this scar?" With the tip of my finger, I stroked the smooth hairless apostrophe dividing my forehead in halves. "But I also think the fact that I was running in circles to her music sort of presaged what my childhood was like."

"Running in circles? In what way, specifically?" he asked.

"Trying to please her. When I was young, I was only a reflection on my mother. She was greedy for the news clippings about some achievement of mine that she could flaunt before her friends, as if I were nothing but a blue ribbon attached to her black wool winter coat. I won the county spelling bee, a Let's Draw competition, and the county 4-H dress revue; was editor in chief of the yearbook, senior class president, and salutatorian; was an attendant in the prom court and a homecoming court; and sang in an award-winning girls' quartet, etc.

"But I still was never good enough, and I lived with a steady drip of: *How can you be so stupid? Why do you have to make my life so miserable? I've sacrificed so much, and you don't even appreciate me. I wish you'd never been born. I'd be better off dead—I'm going to go jump in the pond!* And then she'd rush out of the house and tear out of the dirt driveway in the black Pontiac. Sometimes her rant would include us all, as in, *I hate you all and I wish you were dead.*"

Sam winced and said, "That must have been very painful."

"But what about everything *I* did for *her*? Cleaning, washing dishes, babysitting Mandy, fixing her and her friends' hair, on top of cleaning the church weekly—trying to get on God's good side." I smiled, remembering. I'd sung love songs as I dusted the altar, played secular music on the piano, loudly, until the church echoed with my longings, and then felt guilty for my sacrilege.

"And to get on your mom's good side?"

"There was no pleasing her—I don't remember her ever

complimenting me or comforting me, just pushing me to do things I was afraid to do. Or laughing at me."

"Laughing at you?"

"Giving me a perm and laughing at the results. Laughing at what she called my 'pendulous' breasts compared to her own high, firm ones. Laughing with her sisters at my bare bottom as I skipped down a hill as a toddler after I'd had an accident. Humiliating me—calling me 'Cow' if I bumped into furniture. Stubbed toes were a particular source of hilarity. I'm embarrassed just thinking of this, but one time, she sent me to 4-H in pedal pushers I'd outgrown and without underwear because all my clothes were in the wash, and then they split open when I was playing with the other kids in the yard. I begged a friend to walk behind me to shield me so I could go into the leader's house, but she ignored me, maybe embarrassed too. So in tears, I plopped down on the grass and sat there until the leader noticed and drove me home. I'm sure Mom thought that was funny too.

"Still I did everything I could to please her. I joined endless clubs, won contests, earned academic accolades. What I remembered about those victories was my photo in the newspaper and my fear of having to perform at another higher level until I failed. When I was reluctant to do what she wanted or if I made the mistake of telling her what I was worried about, she'd make a *tsk* sound, shake her head and say, *Why do you have to be so afraid of everything? Where do you get such weird ideas?*"

"When you asked for help or needed comfort, she was instead critical? Or sometimes gleeful?"

"Exactly. And you know what? When I was safely away from her at college and finally anonymous, I refused to join a sorority, any club—I was so tired of all the frenetic activity that had nothing to do with me. But weirdly, I was desperately homesick. That's when I started smoking. And drinking."

I silently thought about those early college days. I'd felt I was nothing, a ghost, a shadow—there were no eyes through which I could see myself. I searched for private places to cry—the unused steps between dorm floors, a rock overlooking the nearby lake. Guys asked me out; I had a certain pleasing veneer, but it covered a wordless, spiritless emptiness.

"Where was your dad in all this?"

"He didn't intervene, and that still bothers me. I think he didn't want to provoke her further, shine the light on himself. Helma, my stepmother, once told me Dad said Mom had been terrible to me when I was young."

"What was your reaction?"

"I felt validated, but I think she said it out of jealousy. To put herself on some higher ground than my mother. Anyway, Brian had it worse."

Over a period of weeks, I recounted my life to Sam, from birth to present, as if I were telling the story of someone long dead. Bits from the past intruded into my current life, like pinches awakening me from sleep, as I recalled a long-ignored and surprising array of my academic and other accomplishments. I'd already lived a rich if troubled life—my brother's suicide, my own addictions. It wasn't nothing. I said to Sam, with a touch of sarcasm, "Just think of my many talents. I can sing, sew, play the piano, draw, design costumes and mobiles. I'm athletic and good at games. I can play a mean game of Ping-Pong or volleyball or Scrabble."

"And what a vocabulary," Sam added.

Maybe, I thought, life was worth living.

I recorded two dreams in my journal:

> *I leave Sara's house where playgroup is now in full swing. Outside, I find that my car has been stolen—someone must have been after the baby equipment inside. I decide to take Jake's motorcycle instead. It's in Sara's basement, which is being renovated.*

The motorcycle sits atop a pile of boxes. I climb the boxes to get the bike, and a woman complains that I'm walking on the merchandise. I'm surprised—I thought the boxes were empty.

I mount the motorcycle while two young men with dark hair watch me, impressed, but I remember I don't have the keys, Jake does. Then I realize I have an extra set in my pocket. I start the bike and leave, but find myself on a street where construction is underway, work on buildings to my left and soft dirt to the right, with machinery and a mound of dirt between. Somehow, I'm stuck on top of the mound with the motorcycle. I have to find another way home.

In a church among a group of people, I've decided not to proceed with my wedding. The groom is very hurt, but I know the marriage won't be right for me. I also reject another man who wants me to go with him in a somber caravan to the snow. He, too, feels bad.

People are waiting at long tables to go in the caravan. I pace up and down the aisle holding a picture of two superheroes, a man and a woman, maybe Spiderman and some superwoman. They are as if frozen, but with the capacity to become alive and life-size.

I must hide them. I go to a very small room with windows, slide them between two psychology books sitting on a shelf. They must not melt. I'm a bit afraid of it myself but mostly worry they'll go wild and frighten all the other people, who don't understand them.

Then I'm outside, waiting for a car from the caravan to pick me up, when Brian goes speeding by in my VW Bug. Chaz, a stocky friend of Brian's, runs and grabs the door handle. I yell, "Stop!" I'm afraid he'll fall and get hurt, but he rides away on the running board.

I told Sam the two men in my church dream must be my husbands.

"I'm so miserable in my marriage, I feel I don't even exist. And I'm curious about what could possibly be in those not-empty boxes in my motorcycle dream, the ones representing the inner me."

"What's your guess?"

"Maybe something of substance that I don't realize is there? I don't know specifically, but I'm glad to think there's something in there at least." I laughed.

"Who do you think the two superheroes represent?"

"My brother and me maybe. I don't know about the superhero bit, but I do feel like I'm frozen in place."

I was embarrassed about mentioning Chaz's build—it was a description of Sam too. Maybe Chaz represented Sam in my dream; he was now captive, his hand clutching the handle of my speeding car, my life, with Brian stuck inside.

Leaving those early sessions, I became increasingly depressed—because seven days had to pass before I could feel alive again. I forced myself to drive home, when all I wanted was to lift the VW off the surface of the road and fly away.

Toward the end of our next session, I said, "I've been thinking about that dream image of Brian racing away with my car. I still feel so guilty. If I'd been paying more attention maybe I could have saved him."

Sam countered, "But you were so young at the time. Why was it your responsibility?"

"I wasn't that young—I was twenty-three. And I'd approved the move to California and the divorce, had introduced Brian to marijuana, abandoned him for months, and then scared him into suicide that last night."

"You must be a very powerful person."

I could see it was an absurd position. Sort of, anyway. But just maybe I wasn't responsible for Brian's death after all.

Suddenly, with an odd synchronicity, the clock stopped and the lights flickered off. Sam stood and excused himself to replace the blown fuse, while I sat idly musing that maybe my newly identified power had triggered the outage and then wondered whether instead there might be a special power between Sam and me, an electricity that overloaded the circuits.

He sat down again and apologized. "These old houses sometimes need a lot of work."

As I talked a little more about Brian, Sam's eyes glistened with tears. He said, "Why don't you ever cry when talking about things that are so painful?"

"I don't know—my tears must be frozen too." I chuckled.

He ignored my attempt at levity. "And why do you bring up important things only at the end of a session when our time is over? Why don't you let me take care of you?"

In that moment, Sam pushed one of my buttons—I was being a bad patient, resisting interpretations, arguing, refusing hypnosis, being totally self-centered. Sam, after all, had needs, too, and here I was frustrating his attempts to be a successful therapist. Here I was, ignoring someone's needs again, just as I had with Brian.

"I'm not used to being taken care of, I guess."

Again, he said, "You're a complex woman."

Why did he say that—*woman*, instead of *person*? Did he think of me that way, in terms of my sexuality? Was I sensing *those* kinds of needs?

As I was leaving, I wondered about the pine boughs on Sam and Joy's front door. Did they celebrate Hanukkah? Christmas? Both?

At home, I asked Jake what he knew about Sam and Joy, and he told me Joy wasn't Jewish like Sam, that she was a teacher, that they'd been married about eight years. He reminded me I'd actually met Joy once, in the parking lot at that nude beach. I remembered Jake walking up to Joy, asking her where Sam was, although Joy was standing there with another man. She was uncomfortable, and I felt embarrassed that Jake hadn't recognized the situation. I thought, married all that time, yet no children. And an affair. Maybe his marriage wasn't going so well either, another kind of old house that needed a lot of work.

I'm wearing a bonnet with lace trim and a matching dress, like a Holly Hobbie cloth doll, and standing outside a restaurant, when I see a group of teenagers rolling my car away, a large car belonging to Jake's parents. I rush after them, but they pick up momentum, and the car hurtles into a ravine.

I'm furious. I run after the teenagers, stripping my clothes down to my swimsuit for speed. I run through three bathhouses containing swimming pools and finally grab a girl in a stranglehold and yell, "Why did you do it? It wasn't even our car, and I have two little kids! How will we all get home?"

Then Jake and I are in a room at Belmont Hospital. An Asian doctor comes in. When he sees me smoking, he lights up too. Jake winces. The doctor intends to use an alternative method to cure me of my smoking. I protest that it's nine thirty and I have an appointment with Sam in another room, but both men assure me it won't take long. We move to the corridor, and the doctor has me lie down on the floor and tells me to take six breaths per minute, which is supposed to render me unconscious. I do it, but resist at the last moment and raise my head. He kneels, bends his head while hyperventilating, then blows on my face. But he's interrupted by a call to another room. I'm semiconscious but see him standing in a doorway consulting with someone. I say, "Screw this," and go to a restroom.

I'm still wearing Holly Hobbie clothes. In the mirror, I see that my ears are very large, elephantine, and dirty.

When I try to cover them with my hair, I also notice smears on the left side of my face from lying on the floor.

Then I remember Jessie's been left with Dr. Goldsmith. I find Jessie sitting quietly in her office. Dr. G. shows me how to give Jessie her medicine without protest. I realize Dr. G. is a ghost and ask her under what circumstances a ghost can enter a person's body. Dr. G. assures me it's only if the person has a high, dry fever or if they are dusty inside. I think, Aha! I qualify because I smoke.

The dream added to my worry that I wasn't meeting Sam's needs. Maybe he didn't even like me, though he laughed at my funny remarks and leaned in his chair toward me. But in my dream I'd worn the clothes of a cloth doll, what he most feared, and had dirty ears—couldn't hear clearly, hadn't been listening to his needs.

That dream also made me think I was like my brother, dead like him, dusty, so he could live through me. I often felt androgynous—was I trying to live life for both Brian and myself? Keeping him alive that way? I had adopted his intention, tried to be a "common" woman, just as he had wished only to live the life of a "common man."

Continuing our conversation from the week before, I said to Sam, "Sometimes I feel my life since his suicide has been an act of penance, living an ordinary life on his behalf. That somehow if I suffer too, it means I'm not responsible for his suicide. We were both emotionally abused. But that might be a cop-out—he had it worse."

Sam asked, "How was it different for you?"

"I hid in the shadows, avoided the limelight."

"But it sounded like you received quite a lot of attention, the newspaper articles—"

"I mean at home, where Brian drew all the attention with his rage, his rebellion. I tried to escape my mother by not making mistakes—that was why I excelled in school, madly paddling my little canoe to prevent it from slipping over the waterfall. And then Brian and I shared the same disorienting move from a small town to a big city, the sudden expulsion into the unknown, and I managed to survive. He didn't."

"It was hard for both of you."

"But harder for him, the rebel. He couldn't bow to authority, and you have to do that to make your way, at least to some extent. You have to take others into account, even if it's sometimes annoying. It's in your interests in the long run."

"And you bowed to your mother, despite your annoyance."

"That makes me sound so ingenuous. I sassed her, but mostly capitulated in the end and did what she wanted. Resentfully."

CHAPTER 9:

IN THE ARBORETUM

It was January 1982, and I'd been meeting with Sam since late September. I was enamored of his exuberance for life, his intelligence, his interest in my mind, his humor, his kindness. He had reminded me not only that I still existed, but also that I could be intriguing, witty, capable of thinking interesting thoughts. Being with Sam was like being kissed awake from a deep sleep. No, a coma.

> *I'm supposed to see Joy, as part of my therapy—Joy is a therapist too. I go to the appointed room and find a big-boned, heavy woman with short white straggly hair. I'm relieved that she's not attractive. But this woman is only "playing" Joy. Then the real Joy enters, medium height, slender, long hair, attractive, freckled. She tells me the other woman is mentally ill but harmless. I keep mentioning Sam—doesn't Joy want to know what's gone on in therapy? Joy tells me not to get in a rut talking about Sam—to forget about that and proceed.*

A clarifying dream. I wasn't falling in love with Sam so much as I wanted to be *like* him, this man who had nudged me from a sort of morbid resignation, the old woman in the dream, to the promise of life again, as his peer, a metaphorical wife. Switching into clinical psychology wasn't simply a whim—I'd toyed with this back when I was still in graduate school.

I told Sam I was considering applying to nearby grad schools, and then asked, "Do you think I could be a good therapist?"

He responded, "I think you could be a therapist."

I was secretly upset that he'd dropped the word "good"—did he think I was really screwed up? Or that I hadn't done a very good job with my brother after all? I could still picture myself asking Brian about his dreams, trying to interpret them in a way that would move his life forward, not downhill. Remembered his notes about people who were trying to invade his mind, even take his dreams away.

Still I decided to start applying to schools, to make calls to my former professors at UC Berkeley for references. I desperately wanted to reclaim the life I'd lost, and so devised a plan to go back to school, leave Jake, work part-time, find childcare for the kids, all at the same time.

I physically shook as I sat next to the stove heater, trying to generate the courage for the phone calls, so afraid my professors would have forgotten me. I tried the deep relaxation routine, to calm myself, and called forth the white light—the one I wanted to hold and caress in an early hypnosis session—and it appeared again, only this time it was eclipsed: a black circle with light flashing around it, which then became all light and then black again, coming toward me, ending at my surface. Exploding and reforming. I'd been reading R. D. Laing and was reminded of his reference to the black sun, an allusion to Sartre, to living death. Only the image didn't feel like that—more like my alternating feelings about myself, good and bad, worthwhile and worthless.

I was amazed that Dr. Craig not only remembered me but said my leaving was "a great loss to the department." Dr. Manfred was encouraging but asked the one question that could dash it all for me, whether I had children, and I made my kids about six months older (two and four) than they actually were and felt the inevitable guilt—would I be abandoning them if I did return to school?

When I told Sam my plan, and about the problems of getting my transcripts from the five schools I had attended under three different names (as if I were a collection of people and still hadn't decided which to be), and how complicated it would be to manage returning to school, he said, "There is time," like a goddamn Buddha, or something, while I thought, *No, there is no time at all.*

A few sessions later, I noticed a new bumper sticker on his green Saab, which already bore a yin/yang decal: A MAN OF QUALITY DOES NOT FEAR A WOMAN SEEKING EQUALITY. I briefly wondered whether he bought this as a secret message to me, to tell me it was okay if I wished to be a therapist too. But Sam was right—I didn't have to do everything at once, so soon. I decided to delay applying to schools until the next fall.

The bumper sticker on Joy's blue car read YOU CAN'T HUG CHILDREN WITH NUCLEAR ARMS, and I wondered if Sam and Joy were unable to have children. I'd talked to Sam about parenting, how people should read *The Mother Person* before taking the plunge. He'd reached out as if to pick up a pen, but stopped short, as if he'd thought better of it or remembered it wasn't necessary.

I talked to him about my children, how difficult it was to relive my own childhood, remembering the feelings I had, seeing my children's pain and feeling my own pain anew, how the words of my mother threatened to flow out of my mouth and how I suppressed them, how I tried so hard to be a good mother, to be different from my own, but that I just wasn't a good parent, having no real frame of reference. My biggest fear was that I would unconsciously recreate my childhood family with my own. Already I had first a daughter, then a son—the same birth order. With my whole soul, all I wanted was to ensure the story ended a different way this time.

I am meeting with Sam, who is sitting behind a desk; other people are milling about the room. I am self-conscious about sharing some notes/drawings with him in front of other people but manage to ignore their presence.

Then we're standing next to each other, and it's time for me to leave. Sam turns away, looking sad, and I start to reach out to stroke his cheek but withdraw my hand, because I realize he might want to maintain the professional relationship. But he sees my approach—we look at each other and then we kiss. He's sad because he has to leave too—some move related to growth in his career.

We drive away in his car, and I leave my drawings/notes in it while we go for a walk in an arboretum, which then morphs into the psychology department.

Sam and I walk in and out of rooms, and people, including Jake, are everywhere in the halls but not in the rooms. I think, Jake won't see or follow us into these rooms, though he may peer in.

Then Sam is back in his office, which is made of glass. He's talking with people about his career move. I'm standing outside in my down jacket in semi-darkness. I see how important his career is and that he feels ambivalent about his move. I don't want to interfere, so I simply watch him. But he sees me and motions for me to come in.

I listened to the radio compulsively now—it kept me alive, was my lifeline, connected me with the world outside my house. Soft rock, romantic, the promise of love. Barbra Streisand's "Comin' In and Out of Your Life" was about Sam and me, the music competing with the blaring television.

Whenever I left the room and Jake turned off the radio, the lights, I walked back in and turned them back on, flaunting this feeling of love, of hope. I turned up the radio in the car, too, until it filled the space, as I drove along from home to nursery school, to the supermarket, my eyes constantly searching for a green Saab with certain bumper stickers.

I dressed carefully for my meetings with Sam. I owned a couple of nice sweaters, gifts from my family at Christmas, and I selected the teal one that complemented my greenish blue eyes, donned my usual pair of jeans, and my boots, my one extravagance, leather with high heels. I hung gold earrings from my ears, newly pierced the previous summer in celebration of having my body back, after Brandon weaned himself at thirteen months. I applied makeup, made my eyes a tiny bit exotic, dabbed a little Vaseline on my lips for gloss.

I presented an inconsistent picture—fancy and feminine on top, but looking down toward my feet, my worn jeans, my tough-gal boots, hard and rough-hewn toward the bottom. A little like my self-concept, good and bad, an egotistic yet worthless human being, almost beautiful and downright plain. I felt anachronistic—my straight long hair parted in the middle, my jeans and boots, placed me in the '60s or early '70s, as if the progress of my life had slowed or stopped while everyone around me had raced forward into the '80s. Earlier in the week, I'd caught myself writing a check dated 1972 and almost signing my birth name, Bailey, instead of Ruggieri, as if I were trying to erase the last ten years. Maybe my life was proceeding backward, becoming smaller like that calculus function in which x approaches zero, nothingness. Just as Brian in his notebook had described his life as "living from death's day backward."

Sam eyed my purse when I first sat down, as if it were important where I placed it, as if the contents were of unremitting interest to him. Of course, maybe he saw it as a metaphor for what I held inside. If I were to dump out the contents, he'd learn a lot about me. My small leather notebook, with the embossed bird and sun, contained lists of books to read, things to buy (someday) or repair, lists of birthdays and gift ideas, and things to do: quit smoking, lose weight, apply to school, leave Jake, find childcare, get a job.

As I sat in that deep chair, I became aware of being mildly seductive—caressing the plush fabric with my fingertips, leaning toward Sam, crossing my legs so my toes almost touched his shin. At the same time, I could hear footsteps outside the room, Joy getting ready for work, I supposed. She was more like a phantom, unreal—I never saw her, hadn't spoken to her by phone for months, not since I'd first arranged an appointment, and now I wished she would simply go away, leave us entirely alone.

Sam was wearing my favorite suit, the corduroy auburn-colored one, and chatting about something, but for once I wasn't listening. I was watching him tug his beard, thinking about how I didn't want to lose him. If the insurance ran out, we couldn't afford to pay. Was he even charging the insurance company? I didn't want to ask, didn't want to acknowledge the business aspect of our relationship, but early on he'd said we could work something out.

Once Joy's footsteps faded, I said, "I have something I have to say." I looked down and paused a moment—could I tell him the arboretum dream? But no, the kiss—too embarrassing. "I'm a little bit in love with you. I know you'll think it's transference, but I only feel alive in this room." It had been such a revelation when I realized I might be known and loved—or at least cared for—to think they might not be mutually exclusive.

When I dared to look up, I saw he was leaning close to me, and I watched as his eyes dilated. Hadn't I read somewhere that eyes dilated when one was aroused?

"When did you first start feeling this way?"

I shrugged and looked away. "I don't really know." Why did he need to know that?

He was quiet for a moment. "You and I both know it's normal to develop certain erotic feelings, to have good feelings toward me."

"I know—transference. But what difference does it make to *call* it that?" I sighed. "As I've said before, I have plans—to leave Jake, return to school—I want the possibility of love and a career."

"I suspected you might try to leave."

"Well, I can't wait any longer for my life to begin."

He smiled. "You're not alive now?"

"Of course I am," I said, "but at a low level of existence."

"Maybe it's time for Jake to come in."

I was indignant. "I don't *want* Jake to come in—he's not part of the plan. Making marriage work isn't always just a matter of effort—sometimes there are basic differences, values that aren't subject to change."

"For instance?"

"He doesn't like to talk about the past or imagine the future. He says what's past is past and no one can guess the future. It limits conversation. So odd." He nodded, and I added, "My friend Sara said I should try to make it work, but just because other people think *their* marriages can be made to work doesn't mean mine can."

"You're right to question other people's motives that might be based on beliefs about their own marriages."

"I've been unhappy for a long time but just never believed I could take care of myself and my kids before. But I think I can do it now, although I have trouble living without love."

Sam said, "I think you can live without love." As if I always had.

As I was leaving, he said, "It's hard to say goodbye, but it's only for seven days."

Was it hard for him too? Or was he mocking me? Why did he think I had erotic feelings toward him? Was he projecting? I hadn't actually been thinking of him in sexual terms; it felt like something more than that.

It was my mother's birthday, late January. I called her, sang "Happy Birthday," and asked how she and Peter would celebrate.

"Oh, he's out ice fishing somewhere, probably drunker than a skunk."

"He hasn't cut down at all?"

"Not really. He was pretty impressed that you'd quit, although we never knew it was a problem. Had no idea really. Maybe you just *thought* you had a drinking problem?"

"Believe me, it was a problem." Without thinking, I added, "Therapy has really been helpful."

"I thought you were just having hypnosis so you could quit smoking."

"There are some other things I needed to work on." I sighed.

"Like what?"

"Well, like Brian's suicide. I've blamed myself all these years."

"You blamed yourself? I thought *I* was the one to blame."

"There were some things Brian did that I never told anyone about."

"What do you mean?" An intake of breath.

I told her about the jackknives in the electric socket, the hanging dummy, the knife to his forehead.

"I didn't know that." She sounded so relieved.

"And I'm afraid I might have scared him into suicide when I talked to him that night—my fears about him not having a real lawyer, what might happen."

"Well, he did seem so happy at dinner that night."

So it *was* my fault?

But it wasn't just seven days, as Sam had said. He called and asked me to come in two days later than scheduled—on Friday, which made it nine days, as if he intended to disappoint me. I didn't know if I could wait two more days, if I'd survive, while at the same time I was repulsed by my own incredible dependency on our sessions.

CHAPTER 10:

A FORMAL AFFAIR

Friday finally arrived, a dreary January day, and I went to see Sam. I recounted my birthday call to my mother and her apparent glee when I said I felt responsible for Brian's suicide.

"You hoped she would take care of you," Sam guessed.

"Yeah, like that would ever happen." I sighed and looked out the window.

"How did you feel about her reaction?"

I shrugged. "It didn't surprise me. At least *she* felt better after the call." I smiled at that.

"And you?"

"It didn't change anything." I paused. "I suppose I felt a bit depressed."

I talked for a while about Jake, how he was gone so much, how I felt I was just a role to him, not a whole person, and that I only felt good about myself when I was in this room, with him. "Because you validate me," I added. "But maybe you're just being kind because that's your role."

He raised his eyebrows. "You feel I'm being disingenuous?"

"I'm frustrated—I don't know what to think—your role makes you mystifying. The lack of reciprocity bothers me. If I could only know you, maybe I could make more sense of my feelings."

"It's hard for you not knowing who I am outside this room."

"Yes, if I could know you, I don't think I'd feel quite so overwhelmed."

After more back-and-forth in this same vein, Sam remarked, "You've constructed a tight case, and your expectation is?"

I smiled, feeling a little silly, and said flippantly, "I want you to throw everything away for me, have a relationship with me. I know this puts you in a bind, pitting your success with me as a client against your possible value system, but I just can't maintain good feelings about myself without knowing whether you genuinely care."

"We *do* have a relationship. Therapy *is* a relationship. You seem to have a narrow view of what relationships can be. Does it allow for the needs and values of others?" He glanced at the clock and added, "Our time is up. Have you thought any more about couples therapy?"

"Still thinking," I said.

Driving home, I was filled with self-loathing. Sam hadn't said he didn't share my feelings, but why was I doing this to him? Being so insistent about how things should be? I apparently was as selfish as my mother always said I was.

I realized our relationship was just as unreal as every other one in my life, a product of roles and just as unequal—I was one-down, the sick one. On the other hand, it was real in a way—his unconscious was surely intruding just as mine was. Complicating things, I could talk about my feelings only with Sam, not my friends. Too embarrassing, and I could predict their opinions, their attempts to discourage me, though kindly.

Back home, with Brandon at a friend's and Jessie at nursery school (part-time, where I volunteered as treasurer), I found Jake sitting reading the paper, surrounded by unmade beds, scattered toys, dirty breakfast dishes, everything awaiting my special touch, I gathered. I grabbed dishes off the table and put them in the sink. "Why can't you help out once in a while?"

He snapped the newspaper into shape, and without looking up, said, "Just do it later if you want a break. I need time to relax."

"And I don't? You take everything for granted. All you want from me is sex and a live-in housekeeper. But if it weren't for me, you wouldn't even have that stupid store."

"What do you mean by that? It was *my* money that went into it."

"I meant the business plan—we'd never have been given the loan without it."

"You seem to have forgotten that I wrote the plan," he said.

I was now wild-eyed with rage. "*I* was the one who prepared all the financial statements, all the figures, everything that mattered to the bankers."

"And I recall supplying the figures. You helped, but—"

I stepped toward him and screamed, "I could divorce you for saying that. You're just like my mother, taking everything away from me, claiming it as your own. Get out of the goddamn house. Get out!"

"You bitch, I'm not going anywhere." He jumped up, went into the bedroom, and slammed the door.

I sat in my armchair, feeling dead, that my insides had been scraped out. Time stood still, paralyzed; the ticking of the pendulum clock was just the hammering of the same moment repeatedly, endlessly stuck. Maybe Sam was right—maybe Jake and I would benefit from couples therapy. Maybe I hadn't tried enough. Or maybe couples therapy would help me to *feel* I had tried.

That night I mentioned couples therapy to Jake.

"Well, if it's brief. But only with Sam," he said.

"But why? I thought we'd get a referral to someone else." Sam was *my* therapist.

"Because he's a semi-friend, and our relationship is too personal for a third party other than Sam."

"I don't know . . ."

I'm with Sam, but he looks different, small, wiry, like a humorless Woody Allen, dressed in trendy fashion. He decides we can have sex but says it disdainfully, and I say I have my period, does he mind? I can leave the tampon in—I'll just be a little dry, but he says he doesn't like "raspy sex." I'm hurt.

We're in the hall, and Joy is leaving for work. She's heavy, with unusual facial features, dark hair, and fat calves, and I'm surprised. I notice my own calves are too skinny. I'm outside when I see a tall, slender attractive woman enter the house, and I think Sam already has a lover.

Years pass. I'm on a street in a suburban city. I ask a man I know where the psychology clinics are, where Sam might be, and he calls Boston University and UMass Amherst from a phone booth. He discovers the clinics have been discontinued due to lack of funding, but I see a directory for the psych clinic inlaid in the sidewalk—a "totem pole" of tiny cement figures, topped by a rabbit. I note the one person left at the BU clinic—Peck, who is there in name only, to continue getting a grant.

I visited my doctor, frightened by the pain in my chest, back, and stomach, which also radiated down my left arm, so that I was sure I was having a heart attack, instead of the lung cancer I'd often imagined. But the doctor found nothing wrong with me, other than my desecrated lungs. My pain was just imaginary, unbelievable, just as I was—a cartoon drawn by Jake, by the doctor, limited by their creativity. Even I couldn't believe myself—my fantasized life with Sam. My heart was broken, not diseased.

After Jake argued that we couldn't afford both couples and individual therapy, I agreed to a couples session in place of my individual meeting with Sam. Jake took the limelight, did most of the talking, and laughed with Sam, while I was quiet, wishing I could take care of Sam. His nose was reddened, his voice hoarse, and his eyes glassy.

After preliminary chitchat, we discussed our expectations for couples therapy. Jake hoped it could be brief—he thought self-assessment could be overdone, become more of an intellectual exercise, while I said I was unsure about how helpful it could be.

Sam looked at Jake and asked what he considered my positive qualities.

Jake flashed his perfect teeth, briefly patted my hand, and said, "She takes good care of me."

I withdrew my hand and rolled my eyes, without Jake noticing.

Sam turned to me. "And what are Jake's positive qualities?"

"He's responsible, a hard worker. If his motorcycle needs washing, he jumps up and does it." I laughed. "Not much to work with, huh?"

I had two unconnected dreams that night:

> *While Jake is getting our coats from another room, I lie down with Sam, now wrapped in a quilt, feel his forehead, and put my arm around him, not caring that Jake walks in and sees us. Then Sam and I are at our apartment. When Jessie leads Sam into her room, there's a sudden silence—he's panic-stricken by the cloth dolls.*

> *I'm telling Sam about my feelings for him, and he tells me Joy is pregnant. They're having a baby in June.*

At the next couples meeting, I urged Jake to talk about certain aspects of his life: the two former women in his life who became emotionally disturbed while in the relationship (one agoraphobic and the other becoming suicidal), the divorces of all of his siblings (as if there was a family incapacity for love), and his parents' estranged relationship. I was egging him on, to build a case for *his own* neuroses, his *evil*—which was sometimes the only way to understand what he did to me. I wasn't the only one with problems.

That night he came home after closing the store and said he felt disoriented, was feeling bad about himself, that he only hurt people, and I ended up comforting him, lured in by his unusual display of emotion. I thought I'd gone too far in our session, pushing him to talk of things he didn't want to think about. Later I worried what his revenge would be. What if he told Sam about my sleeping with my former therapist's husband? Had I told Jake or not?

The next day I arranged to see Sam in a private session, where I told him about the therapist's husband—better coming from me than Jake.

"He took things too far," I said. "I didn't want a future together. And we'd only slept together once or twice. But he suddenly told me he wanted to leave his wife and move in with me, into my little redwood haven. And then he told her, my therapist, before I could even figure out how to gently nix the idea. She called me and said she was afraid something like this would happen and told me to come see her *immediately*. But I wasn't *that* foolish."

"You didn't see her again?" Sam asked.

"No, I was too embarrassed, humiliated. I don't know why I did it. I guess I was so lonely that nothing mattered. Except a friend of mine somehow found out, so I wondered how many other people in the department knew. So awful."

"Was that when you decided to leave grad school?"

"No, but I still felt a little like a pariah." I sighed. "Anyway, my feelings about you are different. They come from self-love, not self-hate."

"I agree, but the issue isn't self-hate, it's commitment. Can you make a commitment to someone? Have you ever?"

"You don't seem to trust my beliefs about my marriage, that it just isn't workable."

"It isn't a question of my trust in your beliefs," Sam said.

Whatever that meant.

At home, I imagined his utter disgust with me. I was despicable, and now I'd lost what felt like my best friend. And he'd left on a two-week vacation, so I couldn't even ask him what he felt. I sank into depression, and no longer dreamed, as if my unconscious had accompanied him on vacation.

Finally, Sam was back. As I waited in his foyer, I realized he must have given up his pipe—the smell no longer permeated his house. Maybe Joy *was* pregnant, as I'd dreamed.

After we were settled in our chairs, I told him I'd been riddled with suicidal fantasies.

"How would you go about it?"

"I'd drive my car into the brick wall of the Watertown Arsenal."

"And what would that be like?"

"A horrible pain in my chest, and fire, and I'd panic, try to escape, but I'd be burning and would die. Fire engines, police cars, and someone calling Jake. The kids screaming, and Jake saying 'Hmmm.' Not feeling anything at first, but then feeling sorry for himself, not for losing me."

"And if you were suspended above and looking down on this scene, how do you think you'd feel?"

"Regretful. So sorry, for my kids at least. Angry at myself for giving up on life, for lacking the strength to persist."

"What do you think triggered these suicidal feelings?"

"My life right now. But also I thought you were appalled and disgusted with me about that awful affair with my therapist's husband."

"I *was* appalled—at how poorly you were taken care of."

"I was also upset by your questions—could I commit myself to someone? And had I ever?"

"I asked whether you *felt* you could. You've actually been

very committed to people and things in the past. To your brother, and you still are."

I frowned. Was he simply changing his story?

He continued, "I think people set plates of food in front of you and you say, 'I'll take that,' and then gobble it up. You take everything into yourself—you seem to feel it's all your responsibility."

I'd never really thought of myself that way, but could see it was true. But more for the bad things that happened. When I felt I deserved the blame.

While muddling through another week, I considered the other information I'd been withholding from Sam, not just that one painful historical secret, but my dreams about him. Too embarrassing, and I didn't want to hear the usual interpretation—transference. But at our next session, I mustered some courage and said I had two dreams to tell him, with opposite slants—the arboretum dream with its sad kiss and the raspy sex dream.

After I recounted them, he said, "They're not really that different—there's the same yearning in both." He smiled and added, "Sometimes dreams hook into reality through unconscious communication. I just made a career move and am now supervising other staff at the hospital."

I laughed and said, "Maybe you'd better talk to Joy then, because I've been having dreams that she's pregnant."

But, I thought, maybe he does have feelings for me—why else would he say something so dangerous? Because in the first dream we kissed, walked together in the arboretum, and then he invited me in from the dark, into his life. Of course, in the other dream, we parted after he'd declined sex with me, and after years of hunting, I couldn't find him again.

In couples therapy, Sam asked Jake and me each to make "sculptures" of our relationship by positioning each other's bodies in space. Jake sat on the floor and had me sit facing him on his lap, a kundalini yoga posture. An obviously sexual position.

To create my sculpture, I knelt on the floor and raised one knee, as if I were struggling to arise, and had Jake behind me, one hand on my thigh, one on my breast, pulling me down. "If there were action, I would spring up, and Jake would roll away like an egg. And then I'd do this."

I rose and walked toward the door, but Sam physically redirected me so I faced the corner of the room. "Now what are you experiencing?"

"I don't envision a wall here—there is a feeling of light and space. Safe and free."

I did another sculpture, Jake and I facing forward, not touching, walking in parallel lines that would never meet.

We sat, and Jake offered his unsolicited feedback about the experience. "What a creative method. Good job, Sam. Interesting, interesting." As Jake talked, Sam stared at me, smiling, and I met his gaze for as long as I could before I had to look away.

Sam asked, "And where are the kids in all this?"

I was speechless, realizing that I rarely talked about them, even though they were my whole life now, because I desperately wanted something just for myself. Selfish, selfish, selfish.

I'm at a party at a department store at night. There's a band, a bar. I'm drunk. I look in a mirror and see splashes of color all over my face. Have I made myself up like a clown without realizing it? Fellow nursery school parent Barbara complains about the guys who have been squirting people with paint. I've been one of their targets. I clean up my face, and then Barbara encourages me to "borrow" some beautiful clothes from a mannequin. I worry about being seen but quickly disrobe the mannequin and dress in the filmy, peach-colored evening wear—I'll return the clothes later.

> *Everyone wildly dances around the floor and on top of the fixtures, and then we go downstairs and do a snake dance among tables in a hotel dining room. There's a formal affair in progress, with people seated at tables in groups of four. As we dance out the door, I see two other nursery school parents in line, preparing to enter and looking staid in their long formal gowns. I think,* What does it take to get invited to one of these parties? What is it about me that I don't get invited?

We were alternating couples and individual sessions, and I had Sam to myself again. I told him I'd wanted to have him in my sculpture, and my kids too, but it would only have hurt Jake and maybe Sam, too, if I'd said so at the session. We would be dancing all over the furniture, using all the space, and we'd walk out the door, together. As I said this, I had an odd feeling that it was both the truth and a lie, somehow artificial and unreal, yet something that must be said. Was I trying to please him?

I laughed and added, "I just realized the dancing imagery is from a dream I just had." I related my department store/formal affair dream.

He repeated my description of the party, "A formal affair." Then he asked, "And would you have attended if you'd been invited?"

Without thinking, I said, "No, I just wanted to be asked."

CHAPTER 11:

OUT ON AN EMOTIONAL LIMB, AN ATROPHIED LEG

March 1982. Jake and I had been trying to sell the store for months and were now heavily in debt to our distributors. When there were no nibbles, we went to see a bankruptcy lawyer, only to learn that if we did file, we might never qualify for a home loan. Ever. Individually or together. If we'd already had a home, though, we would have been able to keep it. Odd. Too poor to file for bankruptcy. And when I sat down to figure my expenses if I were to leave Jake, I was shocked to find we were too poor to divorce—how could that be? All those other poor people stuck with people they despised just because of money? What must be meant by *miserably poor*. But there it was—Jake wouldn't be able to contribute enough child support, and I wouldn't be able to earn enough. Not to support two households, not with childcare costs. Not unless I found a high-paying job. With my seven-years-outdated research skills? My remarkable bookkeeping skills?

After a national chain store inquired about the store, we suddenly had visions of a different life, of being free of our massive debts. The day of our next session with Sam, we learned that the chain store *would* buy our store—for $5,000, the value they estimated of the fixtures and equipment, leaving $25,000 of debt. Less than nothing.

When Jake and I arrived at Sam's, I was shaking, my eyes crossed with anxiety. Both of us sat forward in our chairs, gesturing, stricken with almost uncontrollable agitation, squirming beneath an oppression that would never lift. But Sam changed the topic, and to my panicked surprise, started delicately broaching the subject of my feelings toward him. I was aghast.

"Linda has been sharing things with me in individual therapy, some strong feelings, that need to be brought into the context of couples therapy—"

I interrupted, "What are you trying to say?"

"Lately there's been an upsurge of feeling—"

"Please! Could we talk alone for a few minutes?"

"I don't see why Jake can't be present."

"Please. Just for a few minutes."

With Jake out of the room, Sam sat down in a chair directly facing me, but more distant than usual. Glare from the window directly behind him threw his face into shadow, but he seemed agitated. "Lately you've been sharing with me your positive feelings toward me. Is there some reason Jake can't be told?"

"It would only hurt him. Why do I have to? Why should I have to tell him everything?"

"I've put a lot of thought into this, and I will *not* become involved with you outside the therapeutic situation. I want to see you only in the context of the couples therapy, and I want you to tell Jake about the transference relationship now. Today."

"Why are you saying this? I can't believe this is happening!" I was in tears, in shock. Another horrible surprise.

"Are you going to tell him? Because if you won't, I will!"

I'd never seen him like this, glaring at me, his brow knitted, his voice so stern. "I don't understand! Why are you doing this? I'm already sick with anxiety."

"All of the above has to be said to Jake now, today, because the situation is impossible for me. That's the only way any therapy can proceed."

"But what's the point? What good will it do? It will only hurt him. He'll leave me if I tell him. I know he will. It's too soon!"

He was calmer then. "I think you underestimate him. Will you tell him?"

"Why couldn't we talk about this in one of my sessions? Why are you springing this on me all of a sudden?" I was crying, huddled in my chair. *Betrayed*, I kept thinking. *Betrayed.*

"I've looked within myself, and I feel these decisions are in your best interests."

"I can't tell him. Please. Oh, please. I just want to leave, run out of here. How could you do this?! When we're already so stressed because of the store."

He leaned back in his chair, clasped his hands together, spoke more quietly. "I think you've felt safe with me. Do you know the Stephen Stills song 'Love the One You're With'? Well, I think your song is 'If You Can't Be Safe With the One You Love, Love the One You're Safe With.'"

"I don't feel safe at all right now! Please. Let me tell him on my own. At home. Tonight, I promise. Not here. Give me time to think about this. Oh, God, I want to die." I held my face in my hands, while Sam called Jake back in.

"Linda's upset. I've had a discussion with her about the conditions under which I will continue to work with you and her."

"I could tell something was going on," Jake said, with a half smile.

"Linda, can you share with Jake what we discussed?"

I scowled at Sam. "No, not now. Later I'll do it, on my own time, as I told you." I pursed my lips in refusal.

"Linda has developed some strong feelings toward me, and

we've been discussing how best to use those feelings in the interests of therapy." Sam turned to me, my cue to talk.

I didn't bite, but remained silent, praying for our time to be over. Sam eventually yielded to my refusal, and the discussion turned to other things, to Jake, his reaction to the disastrous sale.

After we picked up the kids, Jake had to return to the store. Once the kids were busy playing in their room, I lay down on the sofa and had an odd thought: Now that I'd lost Sam, there was no reason to stay with Jake. A thought I'd had before—now that I'd lost my former professor/lover, there was no reason to stay with Ian. If only I could figure this out. Was it that if someone loved me, I could stay in an untenable situation? Substitute Dad and Mom? A little relief, this intellectual puzzle, for a while, but the bottom line was Sam was lost to me. I felt utterly dead.

My reverie was disrupted by the phone, and after dragging myself to the kitchen, I answered it, only to hear heavy breathing in response, and not for the first time—a pattern I only realized now. I vaguely wondered if it was the bedridden guy across the street or the part-timer who worked at our store.

Later that night, with the kids in bed, I told Jake we had to talk. I told him I was in love with Sam, that I'd been in love with him for months. And he smiled, said he thought something like that might happen. That people fall in love with their therapists all the time. That he trusted Sam.

"What do you mean?"

"I trust Sam not to get involved with you." He leaned casually against the doorframe, his hand in his pocket. Jingling his goddamn car keys.

"But he *is* emotionally involved with me. He *has* to be in order to do any kind of therapy."

"Well, he's a nice guy. I'm sure he does what he can to help you."

I walked up to him, thrust my face up close to his. "You just can't believe he might actually be in love with me, too, can you? What a wild thing that would be. Well, it *is* possible, you know. It is!" My fists were clenched at my sides.

"I'm not happy about this, but I can live with it. I trust Sam." And he jingled his keys again.

A childhood friend, Andrea, is crying; she is pregnant, her amniotic sac has broken, it's too early—she doesn't want to be in labor. Her white pants are wet and bloody. I move Andrea's bed from a public room to a more private one. I see that Andrea is too skinny to be having a baby. During a contraction I see the outline of a rat or chipmunk, some kind of rodent. Then Andrea's pushing the baby out. It's a boy with a long penis. But one leg is atrophied. It's just a long, boneless cylinder of skin, like a second penis. Andrea cries and laughs, "Oh, no, all this for this?"

Two days after our disastrous meeting, I was extremely anxious, unable to bear the tension of not knowing why Sam had forced the issue. For hours I approached the phone, picked it up, started to dial, only to hang it up again. Terrified Joy would answer, thinking illogically that she might know all. But also, terrified Sam wouldn't agree to see me, that it would be the end. Shaking, I finally dialed, and to my relief, he was the one to answer. When I asked to come in, he responded ominously, "You've put a lot of thought into this?" As if it would be a dangerous thing to do.

In my usual chair, I stared at my hands in my lap, feeling like a supplicant, forever banished from his good will. "I know you don't want to be alone with me here, without Jake, but I really needed to talk to you."

When I looked up, Sam appeared perplexed, as if it were a distortion, which in turn confused me. Was I wrong again?

I continued, "I told Jake everything." I whispered, "That I love you, am in love with you, without you. That you've been entirely professional in your relationship to me." But I didn't really believe that, did I? Verbally, yes, but nonverbally?

Sam still said nothing.

"Maybe it was in my interests, but why handle things so roughly, all at once, with an ultimatum? Why couldn't we have talked about it alone? You had a plan, and it didn't matter that Jake and I were already under incredible stress that day. Why?" I looked straight into his eyes.

He shifted in his chair, leaned away from me. "Well, I've been worrying about the idea of pressing the issue for a couple of weeks. Your insurance is running out, and we're at a roadblock, making no progress. It's not my practice to terminate when insurance runs out, but I was trying to think of alternatives, seeing you less regularly, or in couples only."

"So money is the reason?" I said, with disbelief and some sarcasm.

"Well, I was also under stress that day because of my new job at the hospital. I'm not used to administration. I like to be successful in all aspects of my life, like you."

"I don't believe that's all. I think you developed extreme feelings toward me recently. Disgust or dislike. Or you felt you were being compromised. Or . . . you felt tempted in some way."

He leaned toward me, scrunched up his shoulders. "Is there anything I've said that led you to believe that?"

I thought for a minute. "No." Nothing he'd said. "You've been entirely professional. I actually lean toward the disgust point of view."

"I can say this—"

What couldn't he say?

"—It's not a matter of not liking you, of not respecting you, but I have a very strong need to be successful in therapy."

"And so you dumped on me?"

"I agree that the meeting didn't go smoothly on Monday, and I'll admit to even more—there were other things entering in . . . my work at the hospital . . . You have to realize how important my success as a therapist is."

"I want to know what your countertransference is. I know you really can't tell me, but that's what I need to know."

"Did you hear what you just said? That you want to know my countertransference, but I can't tell you?"

"Yes, I know it puts you in a bind, but I need to know. Why couldn't we have discussed this whole thing alone? What would have happened? If we had talked here alone?"

Sam was leaning toward the side of his chair closest to me, and he was staring. I watched his eyes dilate, like opening doors that I might walk through. I stared back, a prolonged moment I couldn't tolerate as long as he. I started to speak, and he shifted in his chair, breaking the moment.

"I guess I want to know if you feel threatened by my feelings toward you. Whenever I mention them, you suggest Jake should come in."

He looked surprised at this.

"You've said feelings like mine were an ordinary occurrence, so what makes mine different? I thought I should go with them since even as transference, a lot of good has come of them. Can't you handle the intensity?" Now *I* was being disingenuous, using therapy-speak and calling my feelings transference, although I was constantly denying it. But maybe they *were* transference—why couldn't I allow that? But how can some feelings be real and others *just pretend*?

"I don't think I'm threatened by the intensity of the transference. Your crush on me, sexual/erotic feelings, all good things centered on me and all negative things on Jake, it's not realistic. You're more creative than that."

"You're calling it a crush. You don't believe me." No one believed me.

"I realized there was an upsurge of feelings." Silence for a moment, and then Sam looked at his watch. "We have to end now. How do you feel after telling me all this?"

"I've been very depressed since Monday, and I feel better after talking to you, but it doesn't erase the feelings I've had."

"You're a very courageous woman." *Woman* again, not *person*.

"What did I have to lose?"

Feeling a fury toward all the men in my life, how I was always expected to sacrifice my life to meet their needs, I insisted on driving to our next couples meeting—took the wheel of the Bug and forced Jake into the passenger seat.

A few weeks earlier, I had complained to Sam that Jake never left the porch light on for me, that he went around the house turning off the lights, when I needed the light, the illusion of happiness, of hope. So when we arrived at Sam's and it looked like all the lights in his house were on, I imagined him setting it aglow to please me.

Once we walked through the illuminated foyer into the well-lit therapy room, I asked why all the lights were on at four in the afternoon, and Sam said he kept thinking it got dark at five. But, I thought to myself, it hadn't been dark at five for quite some time, so did he mean it symbolically? Unconsciously? That when I left at five it became dark?

Sam offered to meet with each of us individually on that day and suggested that Jake meet with him first. I went downstairs, paced the foyer, and was furious when I heard their loud voices, laughing, having a good time. I felt I'd been made the fool. Jake used up most of our time, but when I was alone with Sam, all I could generate was an intellectualized anger. My rage had fizzled.

In bed that night, I mulled over what to do about couples therapy. I was truly confused. I was blocking progress, and why was I even agreeing to it if I loved Sam and had no intention of working it out with Jake? And why was I hurting *myself* by continuing to see Sam if I couldn't have him in my life? I also hated what felt like Sam's secrecy. Maybe I should terminate. Maybe then he'd feel able to speak more openly.

A few days later, I called him and set up another meeting, again defying the new rule that there would be no individual sessions.

My father has been visiting in the area for months and only has a few days left of his vacation. I feel bad that I didn't know he'd been nearby. I insist that he stay with us—he can sleep on the sofa bed in the living room. He looks at me and says he wants a bedroom. I ignore his look and say, "There's an extra twin bed in the children's room."

Then we're at Sam's in a large room with high ceilings and old dark wood. Two chairs sit in the center, side by side. My father sits in the one on the left. The right one is Sam's. While we wait for Sam to come in, I sprawl across his chair, burying my face in the fabric. I smell his pipe smoke and long for his presence.

Then my father's gone, and Sam is there. I'm smiling brightly and talking, referring to pictures in my notebook. I see I only have sketchy, meaningless lines there. Sam is smiling, as though he knows something I don't know. I thought I'd figured things out pretty well, but it's all been superficial—there is still something missing, and Sam seems to know what it is.

In our session, I told Sam I'd known all along what I wanted, that I'd been trying so hard not to hurt anybody, but here I was hurting everybody, and there was no reason to continue in therapy since I was committed to loving him, not Jake.

Sam leaned forward in his chair. "You've found a way to blame yourself for everything, and that's why you're depressed. But are you thinking that maybe you could leave Jake and then in a couple of months we could become lovers?" He leaned back and added, "Wrong."

"Because you'd still be my former therapist?"

"Yes," he said. "I don't believe in it, don't believe the lines should be blurred. It will not happen, and you can depend on that for the rest of my life. You have trouble differentiating what emotions are useful and to be learned from, and what emotions are good to act upon. It's normal to feel sexual/erotic—"

"Why do you always say that? That would be the scariest thing for me." I couldn't even repeat the words "sexual/erotic" aloud.

Sam quickly countered, "I know that."

At the end of the hour, I told him I'd come in to terminate so that he would talk freely, and he again asked why I always brought up the most important things, like termination, at the end, going home without letting him take care of me.

"But I did tell you," I insisted.

He suggested I come in with Jake next week, go with my feelings a little longer.

I felt ignored and frustrated at his insistence on another futile session with Jake.

Sunday, early May. *The Boston Globe* headline declared "Rape in the Arboretum." I'd told Sam my arboretum dream just a few weeks before, and now there was this horrible coincidence. I'd told him about Jake turning off the lights, and a few weeks later Sam had turned on all the lights in his house before I arrived.

Maybe Sam had his own encapsulated craziness. His phobia of cloth dolls. Maybe he had a dark side, some part of him that escaped his control. *He* could be the rapist in the arboretum.

Cloth doll: appears real, alive, but is unreal, dead. I could see him as a child, hugging his cloth doll, finding it didn't love him back, wanting to destroy it when he couldn't make it come alive. Tearing it apart, finding only cotton tufts of nothingness. His rage at the deception, the pretense that it could love him.

Me, with my pretty painted face, my listlessness, my pursuit of nothingness, my passive acceptance of others' manipulation, like a cloth doll.

What about *his* frustrated sexual impulses? Maybe he despised me for not being real enough, not freeing him from his role, not making him real, so he raped someone in the arboretum. A displacement onto some stranger who had passed where we'd walked together in an unreal world, in my dream.

The more I thought about the possibility of Sam being the rapist, the more convinced I was, not that it was true, but that it *could be*. Given how little I could actually know of him, some evil dark side could be lurking beneath the surface. *Therapist, the-rapist*. Maybe I'd pushed him too far. Teased him. Maybe Sam was the guy who kept calling me and just breathing.

I started shaking and thought maybe I shouldn't see him again. At least I should tell someone my suspicions, just in case. I knew I was being ridiculous, paranoid, but there was still the possibility I was right. So I told Jake, who laughed nervously, but who credited my fear enough to suggest that maybe I shouldn't be alone with him at the next meeting.

I felt a little crazed, but wasn't Sam too? *Cloth dolls*? It was unlikely he was a rapist, but maybe he compartmentalized his relationships with women, functioning normally outside the clinical setting as long as he could act out his fear inside the therapy room and resolve it over and over again. If his unconscious fear was that, like a cloth doll, someone he loved in the outside world could not love him back, then he could at least potentially resolve this fear by caring for his clients, his captive "cloth dolls," reawakening their will to live and earning their love, or at least their gratefulness, in the safety of the clinical setting.

Jake finally got a job as a traveling sales representative for a vitamin company, and they paid for his new VW Rabbit. I got to keep the Bug, no longer had to do the store accounting, only had to stay home alone with the two kids every day and three nights a week, while Jake was out driving that new Rabbit. Only had to answer the calls from collection agencies, since Jake had ordered inventory we couldn't pay for, just to keep the business going until we closed the sale. Horrible threatening calls, and I was the one who had to deal with them, saying, "You can't get blood from a stone" before slamming the phone down. I wasn't sure which phone calls were worse—the heavy breather or the collection agencies. They both wanted something from me, and it was all just too, too much. I thought my head might burst from the tension and little pieces of me would waft down and litter the kitchen floor.

Another couples meeting. I no longer believed Sam was the arboretum rapist. I just couldn't picture it as I sat watching him. That fantasy had just been a way of acknowledging Sam had problems, too, that he wasn't infallible. It wasn't just that I was unlovable.

He commented that I looked sad. I said there was still nothing new in my life, nothing had changed, I still had the same feelings. I looked at him meaningfully and said I was still looking for a job, still had plans for myself.

He asked if either of us would like time alone with him, which surprised me. I said yes.

Once alone, I said, "Do you feel safe now? You're the one who wants to be safe."

"Is that for me?"

"Yes. Remember when you said to me I could depend on your rule for the rest of your life? I think you meant *you* could depend on it. Are you getting off on this whole thing? You can get away with a lot in this room and then you have your rule."

"It's not a matter of 'getting off'—I don't think we're talking about just sex here, something much more than that."

"Well, there's that aspect too."

"I'm *not* 'getting off' on this, I'm dealing with a deeply frustrated yearning."

Why hadn't he said *your* deeply frustrated yearning? Whose was it? "I know you don't want a relationship with me, but I don't know what you really feel. I can't stand that. I had a dream a week or so ago . . ."

I told him my dream about my father, knowing as I spoke that I was *spilling the beans*, that for sure he would draw the logical but wrong conclusion—Sam as Dad. Then I made it worse—I knew it even as I did it—by telling him about my father's French kiss. What decent therapist could ignore that juicy tidbit? I feebly attempted to recover by saying I didn't *want* Sam to be my father, that he was *not* my father in the dream.

"You're feeling very vulnerable. What else about the dream?"

"I felt frustrated, depressed, that you knew something I didn't know. About you, about me."

"Yes, I think that's it for you. There's my life outside this room that you'll never know, and that's very hard for you. How is this dream like your other dreams?"

"In all my dreams I want you. I can't stand that this is a nonreciprocal relationship, that I can't know you."

"I never said this was a reciprocal relationship or an egalitarian one either."

"I know. I can't stand it that way. I know you think my feelings are all projection, delusion, but what if I truly am in love with you? I'm starting to think there's something strange about you. Do you feel outside this room? Do you only cry and feel here? Maybe you're entirely different outside the room."

"And you'll never know. That's what bothers you . . ."

"I don't think you're just a symbol in my dreams. What if my feelings are real, not just pretend, then what?"

"I think you feel vulnerable, that men are unable to resist you."

"That's not true. There have been any number of men who—"

"You're still having trouble with . . ." He repeated the acting-upon-feelings-versus-learning-from-them theme.

"I don't act on my feelings enough!"

"It's about time you were angry with me—I've been hard on you."

"I still don't think these feelings have developed in a vacuum. I think you wanted me to fall in love with you."

"Of course I've been involved in this relationship. But it's time to bring Jake back in. We have to end soon."

When Jake returned, Sam said he wasn't sure how best to *use* the positive feelings I had developed toward him.

Still I believed Sam loved me. Needing to know for sure how Sam felt about me was no longer just a matter of being loved, of getting something I wanted. It was a matter of pride and of trust—in my own understanding of reality. Otherwise, I was simply delusional. Foolishly immature, needy, and subjecting myself to utter humiliation.

I headed to the library, hunting for books on transference and countertransference and felt vindicated by two finds: First, that when a therapist fell in love with a client, a not too unusual experience, one strategy for diluting the feelings was to reduce the frequency of meetings; Sam had suggested my having fewer sessions but diluted our interaction instead by insisting on couples-only meetings. Second, one article that considered the possibility of a relationship between therapist and patient after termination concluded that it could be acceptable based on judgment of the individual case.

In a couples session, I related my dream of a baby born with an atrophied leg, and Sam said my task was to observe, while splitting off the related emotions, the deformed leg that was mine, Jake's, the relationship's, and that Jake's task was the same, except to substitute the "good leg." What a perfectly enigmatic therapist kind of thing to say. Did he mean I needed to face my own imperfections, my own deformity? Or was Jake my deformed leg?

At our next couples meeting, Sam surprised me when he said, "You had a birthday since we last met. How did you celebrate?"

I couldn't recall mentioning my birthday. "The kids and I had a party with cake and party hats, and they gave me drawings they'd made for me. So sweet."

"What about Jake?"

"He was gone." When Sam raised his eyebrows, I added, "He's gone two or three nights a week, traveling."

"How do you feel about that?"

"At least it's clear-cut who's responsible for the children and household tasks, so I'm not disappointed by my unmet expectations of him. And I like having time to myself, once the kids are asleep."

I didn't tell him that, in fact, I imagined myself free. Imagined Sam showing up at my door. Found myself hesitating at night to cleanse the cosmetics from my face, wanting to look pretty, just in case. Arranged occasional evenings out with friends, always hoping to run into Sam somewhere outside that room, always disappointed as I drove home alone.

CHAPTER 12:

NOTHING TO DO WITH ANYONE

Jake and I saw Sam regularly, but only in couples sessions. I was quiet, sometimes boycotting the process, sometimes simply blocking when Jake was present—he always accused me of twisting things, so my participation no longer seemed worth the effort. The lump in my throat had returned, swelling with the music from my radio, the love songs, the love lost.

In sessions, I noticed that Jake copied my gestures—if my legs were crossed right to left, so were his. If I clasped my hands behind my head, so did he. I conducted little tests, crossed my legs the other way or folded my hands together in my lap and waited, and sure enough, Jake followed suit. I watched to see if Sam, too, had noticed this unconscious aping, if he too thought Jake was a pale shadow of me, a robot without a life of his own. A nonperson, as I cruelly thought of him.

Sitting down for one meeting, I glimpsed a fabric wall hanging in the office connected to the therapy room. The door had inadvertently been left open. Or had it? The wall hanging was of a woman, nude, sitting, her back to the viewer, a long plait of hair falling down the center of her back, and I thought: cloth woman, cloth doll. The long blonde hair could be mine, if I braided mine like that. Was he trying to face his phobia a little at a time?

Jake saw it too, and said, "Interesting wall hanging, Sam."

"Yes, a new acquisition," Sam said, then added, "Nothing to do with anyone in this room." Which I found an odd thing for him to say, as if it did, in fact.

He commented that I looked lonely, and I nodded yes.

Jake interrupted. "She isn't even trying to make our relationship work. She's only in it for the money."

"*What* money?" I responded. "But you're right, in a way—we can't even afford to split up."

"You're being too negative," Jake insisted. "If you loved me once, you could again—I still love *you*."

I responded with my mantra: "Love is an act, not just a feeling."

I was, in fact, lonely. I considered my relationship with Jake over, although truly ending it seemed impossible without work that paid enough. So while I job-hunted, I fantasized different forms of murder: a hair dryer dropped into the tub during one of his I'm-in-love-with-myself baths (red lights, scented candles, bath beads), cutting the brake lines of his car, poison mixed into his kefir. Of course, snuffing him was no real solution—there was no life insurance policy, and even if there were, there would probably be a clause about murder. Of course I wasn't serious—I couldn't do that to the kids. Or Jake.

Mostly I just wished that fate, a car or airplane crash, would intervene and thrust me onto some happier life trajectory. I wanted to be *forced* to make a new life for myself. Because the one I had was just "too much with me," to paraphrase Wordsworth.

An abscess was busy moving my front teeth, leaving a gaping space, unremitting pain, and the promise of expensive treatment. I was reduced to playing Jake's secretary, answering the phone day in and day out, and, even better, was given the opportunity to speak to all those friendly collection agencies, with their threats of litigation, until I knew I was a criminal.

The ringing of the phone became a personal attack: *Don't forget you're nothing, worse than nothing, we're gonna get you, gonna get you, give you what you deserve.* Even the heavy breathing calls now seemed ominous, more seething. While Jake was off flying the skies or driving his new car, I juggled the phone calls, while the kids begged me to take them here and there, to buy them this or that, to play with them.

When I complained to Jake—why did I have to be the one to stay home and clean up all the shit, just like always, as if I inherently stood closer to the toilet bowl—he said he couldn't be two places at once, that he had to be on the road making money to support *his family*. Only one of us could have a life? How could I work when already the kids were deprived of one parent four days a week—how could I abandon them like that? Jake's absence was practice for my being alone, for surviving on my own. In fact, it was very much like being divorced already. The kids hanging on my arms, pulling at me, yet I felt so alone.

I *would* leave him. I found a childcare center that seemed homey with its clutter, although my kids clung to my legs as we walked through it, although there wasn't much outdoor space, although it was crowded with kids and toys and noise, although those climbing structures looked dangerous.

With my birthday money, I bought a burgundy interview suit. It had culottes instead of a skirt, and the short jacket with pleated sleeves and Mandarin collar was trendy, so it would work for either an interview for a bookkeeping job or an executive director position, depending on whatever I was at heart.

I read the *Help Wanted* ads and felt as if I was walking through a cemetery, as I discovered all the things I would never be, all the jobs I would never have. Each little square was a death of possibility—why had I never learned systems design or tissue-staining methodologies? On Sundays, I circled the possibilities, drawing half circles around the ones I was interested in but probably unqualified for. On Mondays, I cut out the circled ones and placed them in an envelope so they could age.

Later in the week, I reviewed them—were they still of interest? Then I discarded those whose deadlines I had now missed and those which, on second thought, I couldn't really do. I sent my résumé to the one or two remaining and hoped they'd contact me, while at the same time hoping they wouldn't, because then I'd have to try to convince them to hire me.

To my surprise, Sam suggested an individual meeting with me, to work on issues surrounding my job search. Had he decided to break his rule—no individual meetings—because I was blocking progress in couples sessions and threatening his success? Or did he long for those times alone—could he no longer resist me?

The afternoon we were to meet, I obsessed about what to wear—whatever I chose he would interpret to mean something. And I would be alone with him, Joy more than likely at work. I settled on a plain black sleeveless top, not provocative like my regular summer wear, my camisole. Then, too, the black would symbolize my mourning for the loss of him in my life.

A thunderous concerto, somehow ominous, played behind the closed doors to Sam's living room. I sat in Sam's foyer, imagining him sitting in there, tormented, angry. It felt dangerous to be there, alone with him, so that when he finally appeared, looking pensive, his usual enthusiastic hello replaced by a more serious one, I was giddy with anxiety, and blurted, "Some of your neighbors were sitting on their porch steps and saw me arrive. I was so embarrassed."

When Sam asked why, I told him they were probably thinking, *There goes another crazy person*. Not saying I felt *caught*, that I had the feeling there was something illicit about our meeting, unchaperoned, alone together.

"Why not imagine you're my supervisee, coming for a consultation?"

I rather stupidly said, "I'm not dressed for it." Not for that or for *the other* either—I had made myself uncommonly plain today. A warding off that confused me—did I want him or not?

I did still have my heart set on becoming a clinical psychologist. I'd been rereading all my psychology books, particularly R. D. Laing's *The Divided Self* and *Sanity, Madness, and the Family*, but had stopped talking about it with Sam, believing he didn't see me as a suitable candidate for a role as clinician. I was surprised when he'd treated my goal seriously—*his supervisee*. Or was he mocking me?

When I entered the therapy room, I was surprised again. Instead of sitting in his usual place, he pulled up a chair in front of me.

"Face-to-face?" I asked.

"Yes, face-to-face," he responded, frowning.

He seemed angry or maybe defensive about instituting the change in seating arrangements. Or possibly afraid, not even Joy's footsteps to protect him. He might consider being alone together a test for him, to see if he could still do it and maintain his integrity. The air was filled with tension from what I thought was his suppressed anger.

I compensated with banality, talking about the economics of various job options, saying that a commitment to a low-salary job would be like a commitment to Jake. About my choices: Jake versus poverty, material goods versus the possibility of love or loneliness, the issue of the kids' health and happiness versus my own.

Sam stifled a yawn—he found me boring, the worst possible reaction.

"Go ahead and yawn. I don't mind." I meant it sarcastically, yet my voice was light, void of anger, hurt.

He leaned forward with a piercing look. "Is that all this means to you?"

Which flabbergasted me—it was he who was yawning. But I recouped, "I'm sure you're tired. Clients must bore you sometimes."

I left feeling disappointed. Nothing had happened between us. Neither he nor I had tested the ethical barrier and tentatively reached for the other. Walking to my car, I felt I was even less than nothing.

In a couples session soon afterward, Sam suggested a mock funeral for the store, and I thought it was silly. I didn't care that it was gone; in fact, I would like to have burned it down myself. I wished it had never been born. It was Jake's baby, not mine, never mine, except for the crap I still had to clean up. I said the store wasn't even dead yet. All it had meant was deprivation, and now, massive debts we'd never get out from under. It felt like God was piling it on, just to see how much we could take.

On top of this, I said, I had to clean our hovel, top to bottom, because my mother was coming in mid-July, and I couldn't take her criticism too. Sam surprised me again, saying he'd like to meet my mother—sometimes it was useful.

CHAPTER 13:

MOTHER CLUCKER

I decided to go through the apple box I'd long ago labeled "Brian's Things." This was all I had left of him: his wallet, some drawings, some Sunday school attendance pins, a high school track letter, a yearbook, a framed picture of himself, some cards and letters, and pages and pages of his writings—essays with titles like "The Strong Man and the Weak Man," "Greed," "The Witch," and lists of people, as if he were trying to convince himself of connection.

I hadn't opened the box in years, and yet I couldn't part with its contents or even the moldering box itself. If I threw it all away, it would mean his life didn't count. I took the box from Mom's house supposedly to save her the pain—maybe of discovering she was to blame—but also I'd hoped to find something to relieve my own sense of guilt. Blaming it on drugs, as my parents had, was too easy. Now I thought it was time for my mother to take the box, own it.

I picked up a small picture frame that held one of Brian's grade school pictures. Putting it on display on the table was a test of sorts, to see if I could handle it. I slid the cardboard back out of the metal frame and found other pictures hidden behind the one smiling through the glass. I laid them out, tried to sequence them. I studied the row of pictures, noticing the scars from his childhood battles, looking for signs, for increasing numbers of scars as the years went by, but found no new ones. If the photos could capture the invisible ones, like Dorian Gray's picture, I supposed I'd see him degenerating, flaps of darkened, putrefying skin falling from his face, eyes sunken, his body slipping toward death.

Prom pictures. He'd written me that he'd talked the prom committee into using "The Sound of Silence" as a theme song, and I wondered whether he'd already been despairing, feeling unheard, unloved. I started singing the Simon and Garfunkel song quietly and wondered whether Brian had considered darkness his old friend.

I picked up his yearbook, flipped a few pages, and found pictures of him on the golf and cross-country teams. His pants were too short. I'd missed that entire year of his life, having escaped at last to the big university, to anonymity. When he'd picked me up from college that summer, I was surprised to see he'd grown maybe eight inches, until he was almost tall, as if my leaving had made space for him to grow, as if he'd broken through some barrier that had kept him squashed small.

When we arrived home, I, his cool big sister, shared my lid of pot with him, "turned him on"—taught him how to smoke. Later, my parents' litany was, *Those darn drugs—it was those drugs that affected his mind. He was okay until then.*

I picked up the letter from the psychiatrist Brian had met with a few times before getting his 4-F draft designation. I thought I'd read it before but was now surprised by a couple of things. Brian told him about his scarlet fever and his delirium, how his teeth felt small and pointy, how he floated above his body. Ever since that night, even at nineteen, he felt his teeth get small and sharp every now and then, although he'd never told anyone. I hadn't known about his out-of-body experience or the recurring episodes.

The psychiatrist also mentioned that I was one of the only

people Brian felt he could count on. I remembered the bit about him confusing his identity with mine but not this. When I found his short stories along with notes in which he pondered whether he could make money with his writing or paintings, I was dumbfounded—I hadn't known his interests so echoed my own. I also found a letter from my mother to Brian during his final hospital stay, ending with, "P.S. I want you to know that I love you, and that I care what happens to you." Touching, but I couldn't help thinking, *Too little, too late.* And again, *Love is an act, not just a feeling.*

I also found admissions of despair, appeals to God, suicidal thoughts, mostly from the year before his suicide. With all his incomprehensible delusional behavior, his "craziness," his "lostness," his clear need for help, none of us had understood it as depression or grasped the depth of his despair or that he might be a threat to *himself*. The sound of silence.

It was still too difficult to absorb what had been his experience, maybe always would be. I tucked everything back into the apple box.

Whenever my mother came to visit, flying in from Wisconsin, she would find the one thing I hadn't done right. Once it was that I hadn't bleached my kitchen towels. Although I'd washed the walls, the ceilings, the light fixtures, cleaned every drawer, every closet, and washed the kitchen floor twice on my hands and knees, so she could have nothing to say.

When I was twelve, Mom and Mandy took a bus to California for a monthlong visit with my grandmother and aunts. At the time, my dad, Brian, and I all seemed disoriented, lost in what felt like utter silence, set adrift, as if none of us knew who we were in her absence. No one to yell at us. No one to hide from or please. Left in charge, I cooked, did the laundry, grocery-shopped, and as a surprise for Mom, did all the spring cleaning—I washed windows, sorted drawers, and cleaned closets. I planned the weekly cleaning for the day before her return so the house would look perfect. But she arrived two days early, and when she walked into the kitchen, her first words were, "My God, look at all that sand along the wall. Didn't you sweep the whole time I was gone?"

To prepare for her visit this time, I bought new white kitchen towels, and when she walked in the door, she just said, "When are you going to move out of this dump?" When I sighed heavily, she added, "It does seem a little brighter for some reason."

When she asked me why I was angry all the time, banging around the coffee pot, dropping things on the table, I said I couldn't stand Jake and wanted a divorce, but he just wouldn't leave. She immediately surmised I was in love with another man and said she bet it was my "psychiatrist." I hated her for guessing and asked why she thought that.

"He's the only other man in your life, isn't he?"

"Okay, yes, but it's because he's sensitive and caring." I could almost feel myself shriveling.

"Isn't that his job? Do you think he's in love with you?"

"I don't know, and anyway, he's married, so it's silly, I suppose."

"Well, it happens in the soap operas."

When I asked whether she'd go with me to see Sam she agreed, although she didn't know why he'd want to see her. "Although," she added with a giggle, "I probably should have had my head examined a long time ago."

I fetched the apple box and set it on the kitchen table.

"I thought you might want to take a look at Brian's things, the ones I retrieved from your house after the funeral."

My heart was pounding as she looked through his writings and quickly put them back, until I realized she wasn't really seeing the words, wasn't absorbing them, the bits about the witch that made him do things, etc.

"I thought you might like to take the box home with you."

"No, I don't have room. How could I take it on the plane anyway?"

After a few days, she said I was so angry that I must not want her around at all, so she'd decided to go home early, right after the meeting with Sam. This was a common routine, Mom deciding with each visit that I was being mean to her whenever I stood up for myself after a steady drip of criticism: *Why don't you get some clothes for yourself, instead of spoiling your kids with all these toys? When are you going to get some decent furniture? Why don't you teach your kids some manners?*

When she set a glass of water, wet with condensation, directly on my dresser, apparently assuming everything I owned was junk, I finally lost it. "Mother, that's mahogany!" Even though, admittedly, it was secondhand.

Sam suggested meeting with my mother first, and then with both of us. While I waited in the foyer, I studied the book titles on the shelf: The *I Ching*, *Lao Tse*, Elizabeth Browning's poetry, a book on flowers, a *Doonesbury* cartoon collection. I nervously paged through the book about Lao Tse and thought of Sam's Eastern manner of speaking, the enigmatic statements almost like koans, his almost mystical aura, his references to meditation methods.

I worried Sam would say something to upset my mother, would blame her in some way for Brian and for my unhappiness, although he'd promised he'd be careful with her. But why had I extracted this promise?

I heard her crying, and my heart palpitated. What had he said to her?

When I joined them, I noticed Sam had recorded the session, but there was no time to talk. It was already time to head for the airport.

In the car, my mother said Sam wasn't my type at all—such awful teeth. I hunched over the steering wheel, trying to envision Sam's teeth, and all I could recall was an even row of teeth, a little discolored maybe, perhaps a little small.

For days, with my mother gone, Jake gone, I wept for no identifiable reason, just a global sadness. I took the kids to Walden Pond on Sunday, and as I lay exposed in my pinkish purple two-piece, I kept an eye out for Sam, for any male eyes, but was not rewarded. I felt androgynous, unsexy, not woman enough.

I didn't know exactly what I'd done to make my mother leave early, but I had, of course, always been angry with her for what I thought were good reasons. But why did I still hope for anything from her? Even if only comfort, if not love? We always said we loved each other, a post-Brian mantra to keep surprising acts of suicide at bay, I guessed, but did we really?

When I was seven, I learned what came of loving my mom. One day the feeling was flooding through me. I begged her for a nickel to buy a Popsicle down at Halstad's, but instead I bought a hankie with dark pink roses.

Home again, I handed her the brown paper bag and said, "This is for you!"

She grimaced, peeked inside, and said, "You said you were going to buy a Popsicle. How could you waste money like that?"

I ran to my room and cried. Apparently I was a bad girl, not the good girl I tried so hard to be.

I couldn't remember the content of our fights when I was a teen—I'd probably complained about housework or babysitting or sassed her or maybe I was sent to my room because I'd made a face, as if I *might* say something nasty. The worst thing I'd ever said to her was, "You witch." She did, after all, have a congenital Cruella de Vil white patch of hair that I preserved by wrapping it in foil whenever I colored her hair. Had Brian overheard me? Or had we each arrived at the same conclusion? The punishment for "You witch" was difficult to take—the apology required before I could show my face again. I could remember the rage, telling myself I was not going to apologize this time.

Despite my grievances, I learned to appreciate how much she'd taught me—how to cook, make pies, sew, and garden. She'd made sure I had piano lessons and helped me learn words for the five-state spelling bee. And I was proud of her, even admired her at times—so attractive, such a terrific athlete—a golfer, a bowler, someone who as a teenager dove from the roof of the mill into the Houston pond, a wonderful dancer, who did so many things perfectly. She could even whistle like a bird.

She could laugh and sometimes be such fun (at least around my friends) and seemed to be well-liked in the community. Well-liked by men too—she'd had a couple of flings before and after meeting Peter during the 1960s and even flirted with my boyfriends. So young-looking, such good legs hidden only a little by a miniskirt, dancing legs, dancing with lots of men legs, *I bet I've been with more men than you have, Linda* legs, such busy legs in her boss's office, in the bowling alley, in our childhood living room when at any moment we kids might appear. So many walks in the air those legs took, such dancing in the sky. Hypocritical of me to judge, of course.

I did love her. She came to help when the kids were born, sewed a whole layette for Jessie, taught me so much, prodded me to do things I was afraid to do. How could I hate her when she'd formed me into who I was? When the method I adopted to escape her—persisting and excelling at almost everything I tried—had defined me? If only I could suppress the inner mother I'd also constructed, that voice that said I wasn't good enough, that even my own mother couldn't love me.

At my next individual meeting, I told Sam how sad I'd been feeling.

"Does this have something to do with your mother's visit?"

"As usual, her visit catapulted me back into that little girl who wasn't good enough, who never would be. And she guessed my feelings about you. But still I think my feelings are true, even if clichéd, so predictable."

He agreed. "We both know it's common for patients to fall in love with their therapists, but I think you're specifically in love with me, that there are elements that aren't transference, that it wouldn't be just anybody, and that it's perfectly logical in light of my meeting with your mom. You learned very early not to express your needs, not to be needy, whose needs counted."

"I hate to be seen as needy."

"You need someone who is there, who you can count on."

"I didn't want to pay you in front of her. It was the only concrete evidence of a professional relationship."

"Our time is almost up. You've taken good care of me. You've been very concerned about what I want to hear, very sensitized to what my reactions would be."

"Yes, see what you're missing?" Sam flinched, and I added, "Sorry, I couldn't resist."

Sam had recorded his meeting with my mother, and after she left, I'd called him and asked if I could listen to the tape, and he'd responded, "I'll have to think about that."

Now he said, "I've thought about my reluctance to give you the tape when you requested it. I guess I didn't want to disappoint you, didn't want you to feel let down—I didn't think you needed that right now."

He handed me the tape, and I handed him some money. I barely extended my arm, held the bill by its very edge, and he took it between the tips of his fingers, as if it were very delicate. Something embarrassing.

As I left, I said, "I feel better now."

"I hope you don't feel a *lot* better."

God, would I ever crack the code?

I listened to the tape, discovered that Brian and I were *perfect children*, with a *perfect childhood*, that Brian had been such a *normal little boy*, that I had stayed in the background, letting Brian have the limelight with his cute antics. She wept a bit when talking about Brian. But in forty-five minutes, my mother had invalidated most of my early life experience.

When I returned the tape to Sam, I said, "It made me cry, and I never cry."

"What is it you think led to your weeping?"

"I was so disappointed by her visit. I felt such a sense of loss. I don't know why I keep hoping for a change, why I keep trying."

"Why do you?"

"I don't know. I suppose I should give it up, but how do you replace mother love? I relive it with men too, I know that, but I just can't figure out what it is about me, why I don't elicit love, why I'm not lovable." Except, I thought, there was nothing to me, so nothing to love.

I saw Sam wince, his face grimacing in pain.

"I was also struck by my mother's comment on the tape, that she didn't know how her mother put up with her 'crazy brother Lewis' all those years, that she never could have done it. She made no connection between her mother's situation and her own, how she no longer had to put up with Brian. I was just stunned."

"She's found a way to live with what happened."

"I wanted her to take Brian's things, to take some responsibility."

"And?"

"They're still in this old apple box in my basement."

Weeks later, as Sam and I were talking alone about my half-hearted participation in couples meetings, he said, "In the last couple of weeks, I've felt you were more distant. There seems to be an undertone of self-criticism left over from your mother's visit."

"I've just been trying to be objective." I was *trying* not to think about him.

"What about your feelings toward me that aren't transference?" He seemed self-conscious and withdrew by moving away in his chair.

Why was he reviving this subject? "Oh, you know, the same old thing, but there's no time to get into that."

"No, not exactly the same old thing," Sam said, looking down. Was he sad? He added with a grin, "Besides you and I running away together—"

"I'll admit that from the things you've said, I don't think you're entirely inaccessible."

Sam flinched again.

I added, "I guess I don't believe you."

"You remember I'll be on vacation for two weeks starting Labor Day weekend?"

No, I hadn't. But it was only early August and it was still several weeks away.

CHAPTER 14:

BRAVURA, BRAVERY, BRAVADO

A few weeks before, I'd sent my résumé in response to what I thought might be a fake ad (no employer name, just a *Boston Globe* box number) for a "business administrator" for a small private school. In the middle of a screaming playgroup, I received a call from the director of the Montessori school in Norwood, who wanted to arrange an interview! I explained the noise by saying I was watching a friend's children, implying that I didn't have kids. No children were tying *me* down. I learned the opening wasn't for a back-office bookkeeper but the top executive position, directing the entire school. The interview was arranged for the following Tuesday, only five days away. This launched a whirlwind of activity:

Calling people from the nursery school to provide references.

Borrowing books from friends on Montessori learning theory, even finding one on my own shelves.

Arranging to borrow Jake's car so I didn't have to appear in the disintegrating Bug. Making a trial run to Norwood.

Worrying about what would happen if I got the job: having to buy a wardrobe of clothes (if there was a second interview, I'd be in real trouble) and maybe a different car (unless I could secretly park several blocks away, forever).

Childcare plans, my potential return to graduate school, therapy (Sam)—how to fit them all in?

And what about my smoking? Surely I couldn't smoke in a school.

But getting this job would mean I could finally afford to leave Jake.

I arrived early for the interview, parked on a side street, quickly puffed three or four cigarettes with the windows wide open, waving the smoke out the window, then did some deep relaxation exercises to quell my intense anxiety, before driving confidently into the parking lot.

I met with the director and her assistant and was surprised to see they both smoked—my brand, too, although I politely declined an offered cigarette. I forced myself to exude interest and intelligence, to relate my work at the nursery school to the needs of this school, to ask meaningful questions, to insert bits of knowledge about Montessori methods.

The director eyed my ringless finger (due to my allergy to nickel) and asked, "Are you a single parent?"

"No. My husband will be supportive."

"Because people will call you day and night and weekends, too, and there will be some evening meetings."

She explained the hours, which were longer than I'd expected, and I quickly calculated I'd be away from home from 6:30 a.m. to 6:00 p.m., plus some meetings. I just nodded. "I understand."

They apologized profusely for the salary, only the low 20s. Repressing an inner screech of joy, I serenely offered, "That will meet my needs for a start."

When I stood to leave, the director said, "I'm very impressed."

As I drove away, I thought about the director's intensity, her power, her dusty voice, the same smoke that filled me—we were alike in some undefinable way. I thought I had a very good chance of getting the job.

Sam had arranged a post-interview meeting with me. I'd been surprised when he suggested I see him at his office at the hospital—it appeared he was willing to let me see him outside of "the room," stretching the context of our relationship a little further. Who knew where we might meet next?

I was a little afraid to see him in his office, thinking I'd be too impressed, but when he called me in, I found that the room was small, too small. I bumped my head against a hanging plant and said, "Excuse me."

Apparently mocking its "grandeur," Sam waved his arm so I'd take in the whole office. "What do you think?"

I stupidly said, "It's little—is there air in here?" And then, "Can I smoke?"

He pointed to an ashtray.

I hadn't smoked in a session with him for a long time, partly because he'd quit but also to show I didn't smoke when I felt cared for. But I needed the courage now.

"So how did the interview go?"

"I think I have a good chance of getting it. Because I sold myself. Because I *looked* professional."

"You pulled one over on them, huh?" he said, and we both laughed.

"I'm going to be out of town over the weekend, but if you should hear before then, feel free to call me."

"But I want the job—I won't need to call."

Silence for a moment, as I gathered my courage. Yet again I couldn't bear my feelings—the confusion of feeling he loved me, but that my version of reality might be wrong. If he was simply doing his job in caring for me, I could only feel humiliation about succumbing to what amounted to a delusional state—transference.

Referencing my deformed baby dream, I said, "I want to go out on an emotional limb, that atrophied leg, so to speak." I looked up from my lap, and Sam nodded for me to continue. "I want to talk about you and me. I'm afraid to. I think *you've* found a way to feel safe with *me* in individual sessions, by acting as a good parent."

"I think you feel safe with me."

"But I don't want to be parented. I don't want to be just one thing to you. I want you to love all of me, emotionally, intellectually, physically. And I want to take care of you too."

"You feel split apart."

"A couple of times I've thought you were in love with me." There, I'd said it. And I couldn't bear what he might say or not say, so I rushed on. "Based on minimal cues or ones I misinterpreted to meet my own needs. But because you're so careful, I can't believe you would say such dangerous things."

"When was the last time you felt I was in love with you?"

"I guess after our last meeting."

"What did I say that—"

"But you'll say to yourself that you're a bad therapist . . ."

"The words?"

"It was a series of things."

"You don't want to share them?"

"No . . . the first time was after you said we couldn't meet individually. You were so adamant—it seemed like denial." I lowered my voice to a whisper. "I don't think you want to be in love with me." Then more loudly, "I don't think you want to do anything to jeopardize your career, and I think you're committed to . . . marriage. I hope that's all there is to it."

"You hope that's all? Could there be any other alternatives?"

Was he irritated? He was frowning, leaning forward, his hands clenched.

"What I mean is, you have these commitments, but your feelings . . . I still think you could be in love with me, that you might be attracted to me intellectually. Emotionally, maybe I'm unevolved, but I have potential." *Ha ha, let's lighten this up a little*, I was thinking, as I sat shaking. "And, well, physically, I think you might like to go to bed with me." Ah, that was easier to say, easier to believe than love.

"Doesn't therapy include the woman/adult component?"

"Yes."

"So what's missing?"

Everything else. A life together. "I know I'm supposed to internalize the good feelings I get from this time together, but it just doesn't work."

"Do you think I've taken care of you in this context?"

"As much as I'd let you. But I want you in my life in a more complete way."

"It's hard to be close."

"Maybe it's hard for you to be close to me. My fantasy of you isn't of running away to Tahiti, by the way. I think you're intrigued by my spontaneous eruptions—sudden affairs, leaving Ian, grad school, California. Periodically doing the unexpected. I think the idea of running away appeals to you, maybe because you're so careful and you wish you could just let go. My fantasy of us was much more down-to-earth than that."

"The images?"

"Taking you home with me, having you in my life."

"The specific images?"

"No. I'll never forgive you, Sam, if you're in love with me and you don't tell me, and if you're not, if you've been manipulating me . . . I don't know if I can ever face you again after today if you're not in love with me." Now *I* was leaning forward, clasping the arms of the chair.

"If we were to have an affair, would that be something separate from therapy? Would you continue therapy in here?"

What was the right answer? "No, I don't think that would be possible. A relationship would replace therapy, but I don't think that means the end of my work. God knows I've needed help."

Sam looked at me quizzically.

"I mean I think a good relationship has a therapeutic aspect to it." I leaned back and bumped my head against the plant again but this time said nothing, just eyed the plant, menacingly, feeling ridiculous.

"I think this is making you feel a little crazy."

"Yes."

"I think there are other things entering into this. Something about your mother's visit . . ."

"You still don't believe my feelings toward you. You think I'm trying to manipulate you."

"Not a hundred percent. Do you have an agenda for how this meeting is to end?" he asked sternly, eyeing the clock.

"I want you to tell me if you're in love with me or not."

"I'm trashing you either way. If I say I'm not in love with you, you'll think I'm diabolical, and if I say I am in love with you, I'm a liar and a hypocrite."

"What do you mean? I didn't mean to put you in a bind. I'm not trying to make you crazy. Do you think I'm a crazy-maker? Tell me what you mean!"

"I mean—what I've said about containing our relationship to this room."

"So you are going to trash me! That's your answer."

"You've said a lot of things, and you haven't wanted me to respond. You've said some things today about me that are very true, about my carefulness, being committed to my career, committed to . . . my marriage, and some other things you're dead wrong about. I'm willing to talk to you about it, but we're out of time."

"You're still not going to tell me! I don't know if I can ever come back." I was on my feet now, wildly looking around the room, as if I couldn't find the door.

"I have other commitments," he said angrily, again looking at the clock. "How about next Thursday morning at nine thirty?"

"I don't know." I found my purse, next to the chair legs, and grabbed it. "I don't know." I headed for the door. "Okay! At the house?"

"At the house."

As I walked out the door, I said, "You've still got me coming." I was in the hallway, looking back at Sam who was half bent over and leaning out the door, who looked smaller than usual, angry, foreign to me, when he said, accenting each syllable, "Are . . . you . . . going . . . to . . . pay . . . me?"

"Do I want to? Should I? Et cetera. Here. A Freudian slip." I handed him a twenty.

"Good luck with your job."

"Thanks. See ya." I walked away on rubber legs.

CHAPTER 15:

PERSUASION

I stood at the kitchen sink, beating eggs to a froth with a fork. Two days of fighting feelings of shame over my craziness—how could I be so foolish to believe Sam was in love with me? Two days of deciding I'd rather be dead than crazy—what Brian must have felt. And how could I keep persisting in what amounted to an attack on Sam's integrity? In what amounted to a total loss of my pride?

"You're scrambling them, Mom, aren't you?" Jessie called from the bedroom. "Mom? Where's my Spiderman shirt? Mom?"

Brandon toddled into the kitchen, still in his pajamas, sucking his thumb and dragging his dingy blankie. "Jessie's got Teddy."

"Give it back to him, Jess," I called.

"Baby!" Jessie yelled. "My shirt isn't—" The crash of a drawer hitting the wooden floor was followed by Jessie's, "Oops!"

"Yes, it is. In the bottom drawer. Look again."

Brandon patted my sleeve. When I looked down at him, he said, "Teddy." I was wiping my hands on the towel when the stuffed polar bear came sliding across the kitchen floor. Brandon scooped it up and ran toward the living room, away from Jessie.

I added milk to the eggs, set the bowl down, and looked out the kitchen window. At least I'd been loyal to myself in confronting Sam. There was something he wasn't saying, something I needed to know. While maybe he couldn't tell me he loved me (if he did), I couldn't see why he couldn't tell me he didn't (if he didn't). Unless he thought I couldn't bear it. But that made me feel foolish, infantilized too. At least I'd told him what I needed to hear. I should feel glad about that, not embarrassed. I did feel glad. Standing up for myself like that. Glad.

"Mom, I'm hungry." Jessie looked at the stove and back at me. "Where's the eggs?"

"Your shirt's on backward."

"That's how I like it." Jessie pushed a chair up to the cupboard, then climbed up and pulled out a bag of Cheetos.

"Jessie. Put those back. The eggs will be ready in a minute."

"I like Cheetos with my eggs." She clutched them to her chest, waiting. "Can't I? Please?"

While I was considering, Jessie hopped off and ran out of the room, Cheetos in hand. I set a frying pan on the stove, added butter.

Maybe my obsession with knowing what Sam felt was a matter of pride—the only way I could forgive myself for those predictable feelings without feeling sick, childish, was if he truly did love me. The only way I could feel equal in the relationship, given those feelings. The only way not to feel humiliated by them.

I poured the eggs into the pan, salted them, and reached for the pepper before remembering Jessie didn't like anything she could see mixed with her eggs. I pulled a spatula out of a drawer and started scraping the bottom of the pan.

Maybe, too, it was a matter of being unable to tolerate Sam's silence, of having no basis for shaping who I was in response to who he was, of being what he wanted me to be. And that was how I'd approached life. Ferreting out others' needs, attempting to meet them, in order to earn love. Behaving in reaction to other people's evaluation, criticism, of me—in order to earn a good grade. And, if that was taken away, all that was left was the dust of myself. Maybe it was just too intolerable to face myself, maybe to find no one there. Maybe I was afraid I'd float away like the little light of my hypnotic trance, if he looked at me too closely. That I was only his dream.

Oh, God, I'd let the eggs get brown on the underside. Jessie would never eat them that way. I scooped off the eggs on top and slid them onto Jessie's plate. Brandon wouldn't mind the browned part. Toast. I'd forgotten the toast. But the Cheetos instead? But Brandon would eat toast. I took the bread from the refrigerator, popped two slices in the toaster, went back for butter and jam, and called, "Breakfast! Kids!"

I plunged my hands into the dishwater and turned the faucets on harder to drown out the *Sesame Street* theme song playing in the living room.

If only Sam weren't married. But maybe he and Joy weren't happy together—the affair Joy might have had. And why else would he seem to care so deeply about me? Because it was his job?

Of course, he was right, you could have feelings and not act on them, but did it make sense to sacrifice what might be the love of your life simply because you discovered each other in the wrong context?

I accidentally slammed the frying pan on the edge of the sink and dropped it in the water. A tidal wave of suds and water ran down my T-shirt and onto the floor. Damn. Not even washing dishes could be simple. I grabbed a towel and bent to wipe the floor and then got on my hands and knees and rubbed the floor, trying to loosen some dried-on food—old cottage cheese?

Too many rules, too many complications—you don't have an affair with your therapist, you don't have an affair with someone else's husband, because the inevitable guilt, shame, would sully the love anyway. Ruin it. Because it was wrong.

Unless therapy was over, unless our marriages were over, unless everybody concerned would be happier. Maybe Joy and Jake would be better off in more loving relationships. Maybe my kids would be better off in a love-filled family.

What it came down to was whether he loved me and whether he loved me that much. Maybe it wasn't just a matter of his thinking it was all transference on my part—maybe he still didn't believe I loved him enough to take the risk. Maybe it was a matter of convincing him beyond a shadow of a doubt.

My knees made a cracking noise as I rose to my feet. Only thirty-four but creaking already. Not much time left to get a life. I grabbed the yellow plastic scratcher—Chore Girl, it was called (why had I patronized that stupid company?)—and scraped at the cooked-on egg coating the pan.

Well, maybe it was just transference. Sam as good old Dad. The silence of my father, my feeling that my father loved me best of all, the need to protect and take care of him, to save him from the unhappy marriage to my mother.

Or maybe I was seeing Brian in Sam. The way Sam shifted his lower jaw to the side when he was thinking, just like Brian. Maybe I was trying to bring my brother to life again, unlocking Brian from his casket, Sam from his role. Maybe I needed to know Brian loved me, not Sam, before I could begin to live again.

Or the obvious—perhaps I was trying to replace Jake with the only man in town so I wouldn't be alone when I left Jake. What would it matter, after all, if I made myself a life but still found myself alone?

The damn Chore Girl didn't even work. I took a knife from the dish rack and scratched at the eggs. Better. Satisfying slivers of egg appeared on the surface of the water.

Ah, maybe I was just a rebel at heart. Brian living through me, breaking the rules. Just trying to cut the strings that bound me inside of an intolerable reality—my marriage, my roles as mother, wife.

"Mom! Brandon's standing in front of the TV! I can't see. Move, Brandon!"

I heard a thump. Brandon's bottom hitting the floor? And then a cry. I grabbed the dish towel, stormed into the living room, and turned off the television. "You can just go without it then."

"Mom! Turn it on! It's the best part. Ernie was just going to—"

Brandon cried harder.

"All right!" I picked him up, turned on the television, sat on the couch, and settled him into my lap. Big Bird came dancing down the street in a top hat.

Maybe I needed Sam to say he loved me so I wouldn't feel like a sex object again, debased. But I had often objectified myself. When I inevitably felt there was nothing to me that anyone could love, no substance to generate interest, I defaulted to using my body as a lure, a hook. Maybe whatever his words were destined to be, *I love you*, *I don't love you*, my saying I loved him was a way of pleading for not-sex. A stand for myself as a person, after the betrayal by my father.

Brandon had fallen asleep in my arms, even though it was only midmorning. How warm his little body was. The wonderful simplicity of sleeping when you were tired. Of loving when you were inspired to love. Maybe I truly loved Sam. The simplest explanation of all. Maybe a banana was just a banana. Maybe he loved me, too, and that was enough to explain my belief that he did.

Leaving Jessie sitting rapt in front of Mr. Rogers, with one of her hands, now completely orange, in the Cheetos bag, I carried Brandon to his room and laid him on his bed. The frying pan still awaited me. I lit a cigarette and sat at the kitchen table.

On the other hand, maybe Sam had already told me what I needed to know. What were his words? That I'd think him diabolical if he said he didn't love me—was he admitting I had some real evidence? Or only saying I had manufactured some? That he would be a liar and a hypocrite if he said he did love me—that was more disturbing, clear-cut, that it would be a lie if he said it.

But he'd quickly added that clarifying phrase, that he was referring to containing the relationship to the room, so I was confused again. Which would be the lie—that he loved me? Or his earlier statement that he would contain the relationship to the room?

I was putting him in an impossible position. How many times did he have to tell me he had commitments? How many different ways did he have to say no?

But wasn't I in an impossible position too? Hadn't he put me there? Why couldn't he be more concise? Why didn't he say what he felt? What else could I conclude but that he did love me—anything else could be said, but not that, according to the rules. And I persisted because I knew I was right. I only had to convince him to trust my feelings, and then maybe he'd give up the rules. Then we could love each other. Out here in the real world.

I would write him a letter, explaining everything.

CHAPTER 16:

RESURRECTION

Donna had dropped off her two kids, and all four were now playing in the kids' room. I sat on the scruffy sofa, squinting with intense concentration, writing the letter, everything else shut out, the rest of the world a dim shadow. Trying, with all the power I could gather, to convince Sam we should and could be together. I paused for a moment, saw that I had sixteen pages. Then stopped.

I'd mistakenly thought words would be enough, if only I could find the right ones. I dropped my pen, closed my notebook, and leaned back into the sofa cushions. There was no need for this struggle. No need to convince or to be convinced. To be focused on this one detail that would forever elude me: demanding that Sam tell me, wanting intellectual evidence for something that existed in a different realm, the realm of feeling, to which an intellectual analysis didn't apply. Nothing said could constitute absolute proof one way or the other. They were merely words, and there would always be a way of confirming or discounting what was said. There was no proof. With all my efforts, I'd ignored the essential: that I felt loved. I'd been looking for yes or no answers in a dictionary that had no words.

I stood and started pacing around the living room. And slowly, I became aware of feeling as though I'd risen to some great height, had stepped above everything. The world had opened up to me, a vista. An odd euphoria, a feeling of being in the world, one with it.

Ah, I was thinking of the books I'd been reading. Books on Zen, that had, to my surprise, been sitting on my bookshelves for years, waiting to be opened. I'd recently read Watts's *Psychotherapy East and West*, and Reps's *Zen Flesh, Zen Bones*, wanting to understand Sam's treatment approach, because it seemed he was trying to spur me on to some meta-level of understanding, somewhere beyond thought. His words were sometimes almost mystical, conundrums with no real answer, and I would take the words home, struggling for the correct interpretation, without acknowledging that maybe there simply were no answers.

The unusual feeling of elation, of connection, of unity with the world, reminded me of the final chapter in Watts, "The Invitation to the Dance," which described a spontaneous acting in a world that was process, flow, not something that could be controlled or construed: a dance.

And now here I am!—feeling separate but boundless, inextricably connected to everything around me, that I am one expression of everything that is.

I am happy. So alive! As if I have just been born. As if a shroud has been whisked away from my body, from my feelings and senses, so that everything touches me.

The shimmy of light from the window across my skin, a drop of water on my tongue, the notes of a song swirling in my ears—all fill me with a sense of awe. So aware of my feelings—of joy, laughter, anger; so aware of my body—of sexual longings, hunger, touch, as if every nerve in my body has opened up simultaneously like flowers to receive the sunlight, to receive the world.

I move to the piano, play a Chopin prelude, and the music flows freely from the light touch of my fingers on the keys. For once I don't stumble out of self-consciousness. Somehow I have stepped out of the self that warns me, chastises me, praises me, goads me, and now exist in a place without words, a realm of unbroken music. A new way of being.

After turning on the stereo, I sit in my rocking chair listening to music. When my eyes alight on the tufts of the couch, for once I do not make a silent wish that I could replace it, do not think it is a statement about who I am, do not feel I cannot be who I am until the couch exactly reflects who I want to be and morphs into a brand-new one, just the right style. The couch is what it is, perfect in its imperfection, and meaningful too—reflecting its history, age, the wear and tear of its existence.

The scattered toys are not a call to me to pick them up. They are not disordered, but rearranged—they do not particularly belong anyplace at all. That they are strewn around the room reflects the inner life of the children, their freedom from rules, their creativity, and when I look at the room as a whole, the toys add an interesting layer of color and shape, a certain beauty, to absorb, not correct. Not something to burden me, but to appreciate.

Jessie walks into the living room with Brandon and their two little friends in tow and flicks on the television. When Jessie turns around, she finds Brandon sitting in the choicest location, close-up and center, in front of the television. She immediately sits down next to him and bodily edges him to the side, while Jason grabs her shoulders and tries to pull her back out of the way, and Erica stands waiting, not yet knowing what to do.

I watch for a moment, aware of not feeling the usual irritation that they are ignoring my need for peace and quiet or that they are once again requiring something of me, thinking instead that they're each feeling the misery of their own egotistical needs—not getting their own way isn't the problem so much as their having something they can call their own way, that they need to protect. They can't see that they each would be happier if everyone was happy. What is the higher order solution in which no one has to lose, in which *me* and *my* don't apply?

I walk over to them. "Okay, kids. You need to agree on where to sit, or there'll be no TV."

Jessie, who is now standing behind what has become closed ranks in front of the television, whines, "But I want to sit in the middle. Brandon always gets—"

I turn the television off. "Maybe you'd be happier playing outside instead."

"Turn it on! Turn it on, Mom, please?" Jessie sits down next to Erica, at the end of the row.

"You're sure you're all happy where you are?"

A murmuring of pleading *yes*'s and *uh-huh*'s.

"Okay, and at each commercial, everyone moves one place to the right, like this. See? Brandon moves here. Erica moves here."

"Like musical chairs?" Jason asks.

"Sure, like musical chairs, only this is more like musical bottoms." A tittering of laughter, that I dare use such language.

Driving Jason and Erica home in the late afternoon, I see a huge red orb near the horizon, and think, *How beautiful the moon is tonight, how full, how red, how large*. And then realize it is the sun setting, that the moon is a quarter moon rising in the twilight. The red moon-sun, an apt symbol of my experience—not white or black, but of a different dimension, a different color, combined and separate, one not eclipsing the other. Love/life is within me—I don't need to eat it.

I exist in a different time frame than everyone else. Other cars whizzing past me, honking, driving crazily, as if my world is slower—no need to race anywhere.

The world is dazzling wherever I am, an object of beauty, and I want to take my time wandering through it. No need to strive, because everything I've ever wanted is right here with me, the world suffused with meaning and splendor.

Back home, as I place dishes on the table for dinner, Jake hovering nearby, I see that the unconscious of others is revealed everywhere—Jake waving a knife around as he peels some fruit, knowing I am afraid of knives, attempting to threaten me, although he isn't consciously aware of his actions. I'm not afraid this time, but instead am in awe of the way he is revealed.

I touch the enameled top of the old wooden table, a table I have often thought is not me, because it belonged to Jake's grandmother and I hadn't chosen it. But really it is exactly a reflection of me—my own history that led up to marrying Jake, the secondhand furniture resulting from choices we made. Meaning suffuses the world of concrete objects, and maybe always has—right here before my eyes, and I have been blind to it, looking for it on some irrelevant abstract plane.

The children in bed, I sit in the rocker and slowly thread a needle, then balance a blue button on my fingertip and study it, the little anchor that is carved in the center, a hole on each side of it. How many lives has this button touched?

Who formulated the plastic?

Who carved the anchor, punched the holes?

And who designed the machinery?

Who operated the sewing machine that attached it to the sailor shirt lying across my knee?

So much life has gone into the making of this one little button. All inextricably connected to me, and yet I am the only person in all of eternity who will ever sit here holding this button at this particular moment. How light it feels in my fingers. I hold it in place on the shirt and insert the needle, pricking my finger. A twinge of pain—I am amazed to feel it bodily, from my fingertip up my arm to a palpitation of my heart. I can't remember feeling so much in my entire life as I do this one pinprick.

I glance at the clock, notice that I have been sitting with the button for almost an hour, and smile. Time is irrelevant—I am exactly where I want to be in this moment. I place the shirt on the arm of the chair and lean back. What are these feelings? I feel so much myself when I give up my egotistical striving, my expectations, my habit of measuring everything against some imagined reality. I laugh when I think I have truly grasped it, a reminder I should tattoo on my breast: *The ego and the self may never meet.*

I turn on the stereo, close my eyes, and feel the melody in my blood, sense my muscles forming a smile on my face. I open my eyes only to see Jake looking at me, his head partially averted, from the corner of his eyes, a half smile forming on his lips.

"Why are you looking at me like that?" I ask.

"No reason, just amused."

"What's funny then?"

"Nothing's funny. You just seem lost in yourself or something."

"Maybe, but really I'm more in the world than anything. I feel so good. No one will believe me, though."

Jake looks at me suspiciously, as if my feelings are a crime, unbelievable.

I wish I didn't have to put it into words—they can't adequately describe what is a nonverbal, maybe preverbal, experience, and it would sound so '60s-ish mystical if I were to call it a peak experience, giving it a name somehow making it trendy, trite. Words will just demean the experience, and I don't ever want it to go away, am afraid of losing it.

I wonder too, *Why am I still smoking if I am so happy?* Although with no effort I've reduced my smoking to only ten cigarettes for the day—maybe attributable to the pure physical addiction. It's all a bit overwhelming, the constant barrage of meaning and stimulation. Exhausting. I feel a bit shaky sometimes. Maybe I should call Sam—he'd probably want to know.

When Sam returns my call the next day, he asks, "When you called, you said you were having a 'lightning' experience?"

I immediately think of my childhood obsessive thought—*God strike me dead, God strike me dead*—which was always shortly followed by an imagined bolt of lightning that angled through the iron bars of my jail cell, an unquestioned feature of my fantasized surroundings, and threatened to, but didn't actually, obliterate me. Which is decidedly not what I am feeling. How could Sam misunderstand me so, when in fact he has seemed to guide me to the whole experience?

"Enlightening. That sounds so pretentious, so faux hip, but I'm alive. I feel so lucky. You want me to talk over the phone? It's kind of hard to articulate. Over the phone." The phone feels so heavy in my hand. My lip brushes the mouthpiece, damp from the moisture of my breath.

"Why don't you try?"

"Okay. A feeling of being in myself—very aware of my mind, emotions, senses as a unity, not separate from the world. I think you know what I mean." I feel the blood flowing through my fingers, up and down my arms, to my heart. Or maybe it's Sam's energy transmitted through the phone to my fingers, through my veins.

"No, I don't. I don't know what your experience is. I think I know what it's been like for some other people. A kind of transcendent experience, a coming home from the desert."

I picture Sam walking through the desert, wearing long robes, sand dusting his bare feet, leading me not to something so mundane as earthly love but to spiritual fulfillment, something much greater than a mere relationship, one that can never happen anyway.

"It's more like having been dead and coming alive," I say. I had died with Brian, hadn't I? That was when the long trek toward death had begun.

"For you, it may feel that way. Are you sleeping enough?"

"Yes, maybe six hours a night, a little less than usual."

"And eating?"

"I've been trying to eat more, although I've been losing weight, a lot of emotional weight too. Why? You want to know if I'm taking care of myself?"

"Yes."

"That's the whole point, isn't it? Taking care of myself. Do you recognize me? This is the real me!"

"I've heard people use many of the words you're using."

"Yes, it all sounds so clichéd, but clichés can be so true. It's a different perspective, a reorganization of my life. I think you were just the right person for me to work this out with, although maybe I've hurt you in the process."

Sam is silent for a moment, then says, "A lot of things can happen in the process of moving from beginning to end."

"The process is the end. I feel so different, like I might even look different. I'm a little afraid others won't recognize me, that I'll scare them. It's like my dream about the frozen superheroes. The ice melting, scaring others."

I recall telling him the superheroes might be Brian and me. But what if they are Sam and me? I once told him I only exist in his room, the therapy room, like the superwoman tucked between the psychology books on the shelf, and where he, too, is frozen in place, inside his role, unable to leave the room. And now the ice melts . . .

"You don't have to share yourself all at once. You can do it a little at a time."

"I guess so. I think there's some danger in feeling I've got it, feeling so happy and wanting others to be this happy, and maybe pushing what I know on them, when it's really too much. They're not ready."

"You said in your message you thought I might be worried about our meeting on Thursday. I'm not worried."

At our Thursday session, I attempt to put my experience into words. ". . . Anyway, that's what I've been feeling, and I hope it lasts forever." I fold my hands in my lap, look up, and smile. "That's what I said when I tried cocaine all those years ago. Only this is drug-free."

Sam nods, his auburn hair still damp from his morning shower. Joy would have been in the bathroom, brushing her teeth as he stepped out of the shower. She would have looked in the mirror, noticed the slight roll of flesh around his waist and tossed him a towel. He'd grab her around the waist . . . But when I try picturing myself there, instead of Joy, I can't. It's as if there are two Sams. The one I love (my idea of love), and the other one, who sits here now. "So, anyway, I'm going to take the Montessori job if they offer it, and then in about three months, I'll leave Jake. That way the kids will have some time to adjust. Before they have to adapt to the divorce."

Sam is hunkered down in his chair, squinting with concentration. Or in dismay? Why does he sometimes seem smaller than I remember?

I press my palms together, tuck them between my knees, and add quietly, "And I want you in my life. In whatever way you can be." I dare a glance toward him. "Well, maybe not whatever way. I love you. I want you to know that. Do you believe that?"

"I've always thought so," he says, leaning toward me, looking into my eyes. "But I'm very happy in my marriage."

"I feel very sad," I say quickly, looking away, aware of saying it too quickly, of not feeling sad, but instead feeling disbelief. But wait, does he mean our metaphorical marriage in the room?

"I think you feel grateful toward me."

"Sure, I could love you the rest of my life simply out of gratefulness, but it's more than that. Besides, you didn't do this all by yourself—it wouldn't have worked if it hadn't already been in me." I grit my teeth, frown. The nerve of him to assume he has single-handedly brought me alive again, given me this feeling of happiness.

"I think you're still having trouble with context. It's very important for me to be successful in my therapy."

Why does he always say "my" therapy? Sam as patient—am I a figure in his own therapy? Working out his own issues about me with someone else? "The therapy situation is artifactual. You could be in love with me but not act on it. You're split up because of the therapy situation—the feelings or thoughts you show and those you don't."

"That's true, but I'm very happy in my marriage."

"You've said so already." *And what does that mean?* I want to say with just the right sarcasm.

"And I'm going on vacation with my family."

What? He has children I don't even know about? Or Joy is his family? Or is he speaking metaphorically—saying he takes with him those he loves? That he won't really be leaving me behind? "If you're on vacation, you're on vacation," I say, shrugging my shoulders.

"I'm afraid you're going to be very disappointed if you don't get this job."

"You don't need to be afraid." I *will* get it—it's none of his business anyway.

"I'm afraid for you," he counters.

"If you can still be afraid . . . or disappointed if you're not 'successful in your therapy,' I think you could learn something from me."

"You think I'd be a good student?" A smile crinkles his eyes, curves his lips.

I'm some sort of amusement? "Well, have you learned anything from this so far?" Now I'm playing Sam, turning the tables.

"Yes, something about tenacity, and something about—"

Tenacity! I think of an octopus with its suction cups, of leeches, of . . . Is that what he actually thinks of me? I interrupt. "That's not what I . . . I mean . . . I've been reading these books on Zen. What I've been feeling—it seems like a very Zen experience. To put a name on it."

"If you want to label it." He hands me a card. "This is the name of another doctor, in case you need to contact someone while I'm gone. He's a good man."

"I won't need it."

"That's hubris! Even you might need help sometime," Sam says, his voice loud with anger.

Such an odd thing for him to say, as if, at bottom, he never believed I needed help. As if somehow our roles have been switched.

I jump to the edge of my chair, lean close to his face, angry myself. "It is not! It's pride and humility. 'I do what I am' means I'm just good enough to wash dishes just like everyone else, among other things." I lean back and calm myself, aware of my chest pain again. "I've been having chest pain. My heart is beating faster. I've been smoking less and drinking less coffee but . . ."

"So stimulants are causing the pain?" Sam says gently, nudging me to understand the pain in another way, although I've already toyed with this idea myself.

"I guess so."

"I'm surprised you're still smoking and drinking coffee."

"I have to have something to keep me on this earth."

I receive a call from the director of the Montessori school. Ms. Ferndale, or Marla, as she prefers me to call her, has presented the applicants' qualifications to the board, and they have selected me.

I am shocked. I had decided I didn't want the job after all, and because of that, I thought it wouldn't be offered to me—because I'd come to believe that my consciousness was congruent with reality, that what was inside me would be reflected externally—*What is within is without*. I'd thought that as I moved away from wanting the job, so the job would be taken from me, distanced as an opportunity as I distanced myself from it.

I tell Ms. Ferndale I am pleased, but I'm also considering another job offer. Could I have a few days to decide? Ms. Ferndale asks whether she might inquire the nature of the other position, and I quickly respond that I've been invited to do some writing in the field of education. (I have invited myself to do some writing, to capture my transcendent experience on paper.) Ms. Ferndale sounds surprised, a little irritated that her plans are being disrupted, especially when I say I would need two weeks before starting, but she agrees to give me a few days for my decision, until after Labor Day.

Vacation-from-Labor Day, I think to myself, from the pains of birth. Sam will be on vacation over Labor Day with his family.

Is Joy really having a baby? I haven't seen her since that time years earlier, at the nude beach. She could be pregnant—maybe that's why I had those dreams.

His vacation will last through the Jewish High Holy Days, through Rosh Hashanah, the first day of the New Year, and Yom Kippur. Maybe he does celebrate. With his family, who live in Vermont.

I don't know what to do about the job. When I tell Jake that night about the offer, he suggests drawing up a list of pros and cons. He sits down at the kitchen table with pen and paper and writes, *Assets: self-fulfillment and growth; income for self-support, family needs and desires, and graduate school. Liabilities: personal stress—responsibilities of the job, responsibilities to self, responsibilities to family.*

Is he implying I shouldn't take the job, that I won't be able to handle it? Regardless, he seems to suggest I'll still have all the domestic responsibilities I've always had.

I ask him whether he would mind terribly if I didn't take the job. I know he'd appreciate the added income. He says it's my decision. What keeps running through my mind: It's too far from the kids, too far from Sam. And I don't mean the miles.

How can I leave Jessie and Brandon for twelve hours a day, when I can barely leave them for two hours without thinking their safety, their emotional well-being is being compromised? Too many ways they could be damaged, hurt, killed without my ever-watchful eye. Too many ways for things to go wrong, for lives to end. Literally I'd be abandoning them to reach for some elusive possibility for my own happiness. The job, which could give me my freedom, could cost the children everything.

Somehow the job is too far from anything important in life. It is a strategy for escape, to get somewhere else, but not the place itself. I could do a great job, and still it wouldn't provide what I need. Maybe I can catch Sam before he leaves on his vacation. It's now Friday—maybe he isn't leaving until Saturday.

I reach his answering machine. "The school offered me the job, and now I don't want it. What will I tell my friends?" I pause, the silence an answer to my own question. Finger Zen. The sound of one hand clapping. "That's it. Bye."

To my surprise, Sam calls me Saturday morning.

I talk about the job, that I don't want it because the kids aren't ready to be separated from me for all those hours.

"I think you should consider taking it. You've wanted to make certain changes in your life. But I think if you do, you should give a year's commitment and not make any other changes for a year or so."

"I'm surprised you think I should do it—you're always suggesting I take my time." And why is he telling me not to leave Jake? That's the only other change I've had in mind. Why is he advising me at all?

"Well, it's a good opportunity. You might be able to manage everything well enough, and you've needed something to build up your self-esteem. But maybe it isn't right for you right now."

"I *have* been feeling kind of crazy, flying too high, as though I might float away. I thought you might be able to ground me." I visualize the Tao, like his bumper sticker, where the figure of one aspect is the ground of the other, existence in relation to each other.

"I should hope so. But, in my own experience, I think of it as disorganization, rather than craziness."

So he has gone through similar experiences. Or is he referring to other clients? Yes, disorganization is the right word, a rearrangement rather than absence of organization. "I'm sort of in a different time dimension, slower. I'm driving more slowly in my car, with so many crazy drivers around me. To give a concrete example."

"It's probably a good idea to drive slower."

Does he mean that metaphorically?

"This job opportunity was in my dream. Remember the one where I wanted to be invited to the formal affair, but I didn't really want to go? It's as though my dreams are prophetic."

"Well, I can think of five or six of your dreams in which quite different endings were implied."

I am silent. He has to be referring to my dreams about a relationship with him.

"I'm worried you'll be depressed if you don't take the job, and I think you're feeling anxious about it now."

"I'm more anxious about explaining my actions than about not taking it." I see I have written *SAM* on a notepad, have traced over it several times. "By the way, I think this is what it is, therapy." Meaning that love is therapeutic—what is therapy but taking care of someone, loving them?

"I've always thought you did."

Enigmatic again. Using "always" as if he is a god or something.

He asks, "Did you have any reactions to our meeting Thursday?"

"I think you gave me exactly what I asked for, a whack on the head."

I hear his indrawn breath.

I say, "I mean the hubris thing. I knew I was getting carried away with myself. Why else would I be so angry when you mentioned it? You brought me more down to earth."

"We can speak in more depth when I return."

After the Labor Day weekend, I call the school and decline the job. I shake as I refer to a piece of paper in my hand, where I've jotted down my reasons. Ms. Ferndale seems distracted—her plans have gone awry—and is, perhaps, already visualizing calling the next best candidate.

I call my references, feeling foolish about declining the job after involving their efforts in getting it, but everybody oozes understanding the minute I mention my children, their needs.

My life falls back into a familiar place—Jessie in nursery school, Brandon in playgroups, me finding time for myself by arranging babysitting exchanges.

Later in the week, I have my teeth cleaned at the periodontist's. I happily socialize with the hygienist and focus on achieving an egoless state, on trusting her. But later in the day, I notice one of my lower teeth has sharp, exposed edges, as if it has been broken. I had been too relaxed, hadn't given the necessary cues that would have signaled the hygienist to be more careful. But when I go back in, the periodontist shows me the X-rays taken before the cleaning—the tooth had been broken long before. I feel foolish.

Jake and I are at a hospital—St. Elizabeth's or Mount Auburn, because the teeth in the upper left part of my mouth keep falling out. I repeatedly try to push them back in place so they will remain viable, but they eventually disintegrate. My gums become soft and pliable, and tissue begins to fall out in patches. Jake is complaining about the cost of the visit, and I yell, "I am not going to go toothless just because you don't want to spend the money!"

I'm having trouble speaking and holding my teeth and gums in place. A nurse hands me a napkin and I let it all fall out—there is nothing I can do to put it all back together the same way it was. She asks whether I have checked in, and explains that in order to be treated, I must call home to show I know my own number. I think it's funny, because if I'm at the hospital, nobody's at home. I ask, "You mean I have to go back to 'go'?" The woman says yes.

In the parking lot, Jake suggests maybe I should go to a different hospital, where I might be better cared for—it's only a little farther away from home. I worry that it's too far away from the kids.

The cellar is musty and dark, and the elderly woman taps her toe and hugs her miniature poodle to her powdery cheek, as she waits for my decision about the desk.

"It was my son Ted's. Long gone now, married with . . . Well, he was married, but now, anyway, he swears he doesn't want it, his boys just hate school, well, you know boys, anyway they think they do, and I just thought someone . . . Only the drawers, I suppose, are a drawback."

I yank at the top drawer again with one hand.

The woman says, "I suppose there must be a key. In the drawer maybe."

As I study the old oak desk, wondering where exactly I'll put such a large, unsightly piece of furniture, marred as it is with coffee rings and peeling veneer, I unconsciously touch my finger to my earlobe to twist the emerald stud, and when I find it absent, think I might cry. Such a little thing to want—to wear earrings—and how much I long for those little decorations to my self-concept. But I'm allergic to metal—probably a nickel alloy is the culprit, my doctor had said as he wrote me a prescription for cortisone cream.

The old woman steps near, peers up at me. "You don't like it? Only five dollars, then. If you cart it away." I try the drawer again. "Those drawers," she says, and shakes her head. "Cost us a lot more than that."

I touch my ear again. My dream about having large, dirty ears. Prophetic again. Metaphorical—not hearing what Sam is saying. He'll get a kick out of that association—I'll have to remember to tell him when he is back. From his vacation. With his family.

Donna, Jason and Erica's mother, who has backed her station wagon into the old woman's driveway just in case, walks down the cement steps from the bulkhead. "That's a perfect desk, Linda."

"Except for the drawers. Which don't open."

"We'll get them open, one way or another," Donna says as she jerks one of the drawers.

I don't really need those earrings or a new car or any new clothes now that I'm not taking that fancy job that Sam had said "would have paid too much anyway." Whatever that meant—had he meant it ironically? That the salary was inconsistent with my inferior self-image? Or instead, that too much was at risk?

I don't need earrings to write and draw, to translate my new vision of reality onto paper, and that's what I intend to do. I am just a simple person, and now someone with a goal, and the goal is the thing, not the flash of gems to frame my face. But I will need a desk.

"I'll take it!" I say, and as if they have been holding their breath, frozen in place, and are now released, the old woman sighs, while Donna takes one end of the desk and tugs.

As Donna and I tip the desk to fit it through the bulkhead door, the drawers fall open—a good sign.

The same day I bring home my desk, I receive another of what have become frequent crank phone calls. Most involve silence followed by the caller hanging up. Once, earlier in the summer, a man said he was a secret admirer, and when he called me by name, I said angrily that I had "no time for any secret admirers" and slammed the phone down, thinking of that Zen koan, *If you love, love openly*.

Often the calls come at 5:45 p.m., just after Jake returns to the store after his dinner break, so maybe it's a neighbor who can see him leave. Maybe the wheelchair-bound man with MS who lives across the street. Or maybe the fellow who works at the store, who knows when Jake will be en route. At one time, I thought maybe it was Sam, who also knows Jake's schedule, who might love me but can't say it and so could be reduced to silent calls, to secrets.

So strange—maybe a telephone malfunction? But the frequency of the calls makes it seem unlikely. I recall the fuses blowing in Sam's house and my impression from Sam's behavior that it was a meaningful event, as if some power is generated by the two of us coming together in the same room. Maybe there are psychic energies that no one understands, that most people attribute to superstition, but that still exist despite the limitations of our own primitive minds to comprehend them.

Maybe I am personally creating the ringing of the phones, wanting so much to connect with Sam.

I recall my dream in which, paradoxically, I am asked to phone home, to call my own number, as proof of identity, when, of course, I am not there to answer.

Or a further stretch: Can it be someone reaching out to me from another dimension? From the spirit world? Brian? Is it a sign?

After many rings, I finally pick up the receiver. I can hear heavy breathing, the sounds of masturbation, or the last gasps of someone dying. I can't hang up this time—I want to confront him—so I say, "If you're so crazy about me, why won't you tell me your name?"

The man responds in a deep voice, "I *will*."

I hang up immediately, afraid to hear his name, afraid I've taken it too far, that whoever it was might come for me. I'm frightened.

Jake is out of town, and I imagine it's him calling me, and in his sexual frustration, masturbating. Imagine that he has gone mad and wants to hurt me.

Or Sam—if he loves me, he too must be frustrated. It could have been him, but the voice sounded more like Jake's. I am terrified.

When Jake calls that night, he tells the kids he has a surprise for them and a special surprise for me. A Saturday night special, I fear. He will come home with a gun to kill me. The kids will be murdered next, getting something a little less special, but still guilty by reason of being half-me.

Of course I am being silly, aren't I? But I can't quite shake the feeling. The man's *I will* runs through my mind: Godlike will or the Devil's will. Some power that someone wants to exert over me, that I am denying, resisting. His name: I WILL.

Other nursery school mothers and I meet at Susan's house to review the carpool schedule I've designed, and the women rave about how well I've organized it so that it works for everyone's schedule. When I mention some of my ideas for the nursery school, I am surprised and a little amused when the women excitedly tell me they haven't thought about it quite like that before, what interesting ideas—I should talk to the board. As if I am a wise person, as if my peak experience has changed me. It isn't just my imagination.

But at home, the fear creeps back. It is 5:00 p.m. and I am terrified. Jake will be returning that night, and I don't know what to do, whether to believe my intuition and run away with the kids to a friend's house, or whether to stay, to assume I am just being paranoid.

I've been cruel to him, refusing to work on our marriage, turning my back to him in bed, being generally dismissive, clearly wanting him gone, and he hasn't reacted. Maybe his anger is all amassed inside, ready to explode with murderous force. What to do?

I wander through the house, trying to think whether to hide, where to hide. Whether to have something available for use as a weapon if it should be true.

I am panicky, can't think straight.

Of course, he wishes to murder me. He reveals his unconscious all the time—brandishing those knives, murdering my feelings by turning off the lights, turning down the heat, turning off the radio. He hasn't been conscious of it, but it has built in him slowly, the urge to violence, and now he has lost his mind and will finally kill me, kill the children. Maybe himself.

He is at the door.

I am in the kitchen.

I tell the kids to stay with me, but they resist and run to him, yelling, "Treat! Treat!" He hands them a bag and they run into the kitchen with it, show me the doughnuts inside, cider jelly doughnuts.

But there is still my special something.

Jake comes into the room, his hand in a bag. He will pull out a gun, I am sure of it, and I back away from him, clutch my shirt, my heart beating so hard—oh, what can I do?

But no, it is only a jar of apple cider jelly. I sigh deeply. It's appropriate, his bringing these things.

I've been wrong. The murdering is expressed metaphorically. Apple cider doughnuts, apple cider jelly: the serpent offering the apple to Eve. But an adulteration of this—tainted apples, all mixed up with other things, a defilement of the event in the Garden of Eden.

I refuse to eat the doughnuts.

I put the jelly in the refrigerator. I will not eat that either.

His offerings, a defilement.

PART IV:

THE SUN, THE MOON, AND THE DEVIL, 1982

CHAPTER 17:

A STRANGE CONJUNCTION OF INFLUENCES

Thursday, September 23, 1982, the autumnal equinox, when night almost equals day. I am driving down Mount Auburn Street on my way to Sam's, for our first meeting since his vacation, thinking about Jake lying now in the dental chair, and how typical it is for him to decide he should go to the dentist because I have dental problems—he cannot even allow me to have gum problems all to myself—when someone blasts a horn, and I notice how erratically other cars are driving, whizzing by, weaving in and out as if they are being chased. So I slow down further, look in the rearview mirror for the pursuer and am only dizzied by the onslaught of more cars coming at me from behind, more horns honking. When I look forward again, I see construction underway, a mound of earth on one side of the street and machinery on the other, and I laugh aloud. God, how like my dream of being stuck on a mound of dirt in a construction area and needing to find another way home.

As I approach Sam's house, I find more construction on the street, barring my way. It is not merely like my dream, it is my dream unfolding, and I panic—maybe Sam's house is no longer there, maybe all of reality is changed. I pull over when I see a construction worker, ask whether there is a way I can get through, and then detour around the block. As in my dream, I must find another way. I creep slowly up Sam's street, looking left and right to see what might have changed, wondering if this is actually his street or just some convincing stage set mimicking my dream.

His green Saab is parked on the street facing me. I pull over before passing his driveway and park in front of the neighbor's house so my white Bug faces his Saab. Face-to-face, I think with amusement. Joy's blue car is in the driveway, its nose out toward the street, as if ready to leave (yes, please), and farther down the driveway there is a yellow car I haven't seen before, also pointing toward the street, bearing Virginia license plates. The color of the sun, of light, Virgin-ia—Sam's and my car? The car ready, Sam waits for me, to become as a virgin—it is only appropriate that we should go to Virginia in it or into a metaphorically pure state.

I walk into the foyer and pace. A woman, a client, descends from upstairs, and says, "It's cold in here today."

Sam is cold today, I think, and I shiver. I feel a cold power from upstairs.

I am standing near his bookcase, and I peer up the stairs and see Sam without his knowing. He goes into the bedroom, looks, and then shuts the door, checks other doors and closes them. Why has he checked his bedroom? Readying things—oh, God—or blocking the unallowable from view? He approaches the stairs, I move out of sight, and then he invites me to come up.

"How was your vacation?" I ask.

"Great!"

I think he means "grate," as I often use the word, facetiously. Grating, raspy.

"Good!"

I tell him about my infected ears, and sure enough, he seems to believe the site of infection is meaningful, that my hearing has been affected, so I add, "I mean my earlobes, from my pierced earrings. I had to stop wearing my wedding ring, too, because of a rash." I laugh and look at him out of the corner of my eye. "Allergic to metal, I guess."

"Allergic to metal!"

I wonder why he thinks this meaningful—meddle? Mettle? "Even 24k gold. Maybe it's the nickel alloy. I keep wondering if coffee and cigarettes have changed my body chemistry to a more acid state, so that it leaches the metal or something."

I tell him of the repeated phone calls, and recount the *I will* phone call verbatim, adding that the ragged breath sounded like someone masturbating or someone dying, and how scared I was, how it sounded like Jake's voice. "I haven't satisfied him sexually in a long time, so it could have been him."

I look up at Sam, and to my wonder, he has sprouted horns. He leans forward, angry, intense, like the Devil. For a moment, all I can do is stare, yet I am not afraid. The horns are the visual expression of his anger about my experience, that someone would threaten me like that. He is my ally, isn't he?

"But I also thought it might have been you."

His eyes radiate intensity.

I add, "It would have been perfectly logical."

"You *believed* it could be me?"

"I didn't really believe it, no."

"But you *felt* it could be me?" He is perched on the edge of his chair, his hands clamped against the chair arms. I watch his fingers turn white, and then look at my own hands clasped together in my lap.

"Yes, it would be perfectly understandable. If you were in love with me or at least had erotic feelings toward me, then I haven't satisfied you either. But I really believed it was Jake."

I tell him about Jake's phone call and my fear that Jake was planning to murder me and the kids, but that instead he'd brought apple cider doughnuts and jelly. How I still think he displays his unconscious wish to murder me in various ways.

Sam's horns recede. I cannot look at him closely because an aura of brightness surrounding him hurts my eyes. He is so intense today. When I look at him next, his face appears sexual, like a woman's genitals, with his hair and beard framing his face. I myself, with my hair parted down the middle and drawn together with an elastic band, must look like a sperm. There we are, face-to-face, with Sam reversed as in the Tao, the 69 position. And, I think, we both know not only that we are locked into this sexual appearance, but also that it cannot be spoken of. Both are aware of how difficult it is to bear without acknowledging its strangeness, as if we are puppets, costumed by someone greater, powerless even to acknowledge that this experience is mutual.

"I think you're feeling very bad about not having taken that job at the school," Sam says, pushing the words out as if he is struggling to create the appearance of a normal therapy session.

"No, actually. I'm planning to do some writing about some ideas that have come out of my . . . you know, my peak experience, and I'm very excited about it. I know it sounds grandiose, but I think there's some truth in the ideas."

I look out the window just as an orange maple leaf blows against the glass, clings for a moment, then falls. I shake my head—what I do not want to happen, a falling away of the beauty, the good feelings.

"But I keep coming back to the idea that even if you are your own true self, and you've learned to love yourself, what difference does it make if still no one loves you? Then I feel like dying." I take a deep breath. "Just like dying. That's why it's so important for me to know how you feel." As I say it, knowing it's useless, I feel a creeping humiliation spread through my body like a flush of heat. "There really is no one else who cares, except maybe the kids, and I can't hold them responsible for my happiness. I can't stay alive just for them."

"You're still forgetting context," Sam says, pulling a stock phrase out of his therapist's hat.

"No, I'm not. Therapy is in the world—it's not just 'pretend.' I think therapy is love, and that's what I meant when I said on the phone that I thought this was therapy. I think I'll die if this isn't really love." I am aware of my own melodrama, but still—how can he continue to believe that secrecy is therapeutic? How can you trust someone you aren't even allowed to know?

"Do you think you can last until our next session? Our time is up for today." He smiles.

How dare he be amused. Okay, so maybe it sounded like hyperbole. But I meant what I said.

As I leave the house, I notice Joy's car is gone. Passing his house in order to turn around on the dead-end street, I see Sam in my rearview mirror, getting into his car, removing the keys apparently, and when I turn around, he waves to me before returning to the house. He is showing me something: removing the keys from his car—leaving his individual life for ours—Sam's and mine. He is becoming virginal, removing the keys, the symbolic sexuality of keys in the ignition—he will no longer sleep with his wife. The yellow car awaits—our car.

I smile and wave, acknowledging the message. He has left his house, has walked out the door with me, telling me he will be there on the other side if I walk out the door, leave therapy. By taking the keys out of the ignition, he is also saying he isn't going anywhere—as if somehow the real way to leave is to stay. The real world will be reordered by staying where he doesn't belong—the world will reorganize around him until a new harmony is found. What is within is without; what is inside is outside. He will stay to leave. Jewish High Holy Days. He will be vacating, fasting for the holiday. And while he stays, I am in control; I am the one driving. It is up to me—I am in charge, and he is counting on me.

At the nursery school that night, another parent, Susan, sits next to me, whispering complaints in the form of questions, as if she can own them only with my agreement. We sit on tiny chairs, our knees approaching our chins. I discreetly munch an apple. I was amused earlier to see the plate of apples, an aberration among the customary fancy desserts, as if they were drawn there by the imagery floating through my mind. Susan talks into my ear, while I eat, thinking that it's okay to eat this apple, this symbolic apple of knowledge, in its pure state, not cooked and defiled by its conjunction with other ingredients, like the cider jelly Jake gave me.

When I see the class list, the children's names separated into boys and girls, I wave my hand until the director acknowledges me. I say maybe it's minor, but I think separate lists subtly encourage differential treatment, which isn't consistent with the philosophy of the school.

Other parents nod and say they agree until the director apologizes. When a special committee is to be formed, one of the men suggests I should be on it—I have good ideas. But when the list of usual committees is handed out, I can't find my name anywhere, even though every parent is expected to be on one. I am bewildered by this omission.

After the meeting, I ask the president, Barbara, another parent, about it, and she says it must be a typographical error. But the director overhears and says it was decided I'd contributed so much last year as treasurer that I didn't need to work on a committee this year.

Of course it is a subterfuge. Just a few months before, the director had raved about my financial work, but somehow she's now feeling threatened by my influence. I leave, feeling rejected, hurt. It is like my dream, in which I'm not invited to the formal affair, to the tables of four. No job, no love, no nursery school work, as if I am systematically being excluded from all of life.

The evening seems bizarre. Is it the impact of the autumnal equinox? Some disjunction in the movement of the seasons?

Tomorrow is the moon's first quarter, the balance of black and white, shadow and light, the Tao. And it is Jewish High Holy Days. How often do all of these influences coincide? Is this a particularly strange conjunction?

I lie in bed, unable to sleep. Jake lies in blackness next to me, a phantom mound of darkness. I face away from him, staring out the window, the shade half-drawn only, the window open, the open portion of a casket. I must have some light in this room or I will die here.

I try to make my thoughts travel along the geographic lines from my window to Sam's house in Belmont. Does he catch my thoughts? Do they float into his mind as I send them? *Please love me.* There's no way out of this room, only this little light, a string of hope passing through the tiny squares of window screen. Layers and layers of entrapment, Jake, the children, debts, lost time, smoke, on and on. No one knows I am here, dying, dying. *Please let me out. Please, God, don't let me die here in this emptiness.* Finally, I sleep.

CHAPTER 18:

WHAT IS WITHIN IS WITHOUT

Friday, 9/24. I awaken very early, at sunrise. I have the house to myself, everyone else still asleep. I put the kettle on and muse about my meeting with Sam yesterday. He is more powerful than I have believed. His horns, his cold anger in defense of me. His amusement, asking whether I can last until next week, as if I will live forever, am powerful too. He discounts my need of him—we are peers. He is trying to tell me something, something I must discover about our relationship, about this time of year, something special about the conjunction of influences. Perhaps all my life has led up to this—something I am to do, a meaning to my life that extends beyond the personal.

I get my notebook, stir my cup of coffee, sit at the kitchen table, and try to decipher meanings that perhaps have been obscured through intervening history.

I write: *Although everything is meaningful, the meanings have been confused over time, lost, as if the Tower of Babel had resulted not only in different languages, but in confusion within each language itself, and not only language, but numerical systems, calendar systems.*

Maybe the trick is to discover the true meanings by observing the details of the concrete world, by reordering, rearranging them into their original forms. Anagrams to be solved. Math functions to be understood from a new perspective.

Jake walks into the kitchen, and immediately I close my notebook, feeling a flush of embarrassment. He stands there in his underwear, looking first at me, then at the closed notebook, and then back at me, with a frown. "Up awful early, aren't you?"

"You too." I sit very still, waiting for him to leave.

He won't understand my work—it must not be revealed to him. Too early—he is not ready for this. Most of the world is not, for that matter. I get up and slide my notebook into a drawer, after seeing his suspicious look. Maybe he has been here all along, infiltrating my life to prevent me from this work. From that which I have been called to perform? Jake, a sinister overseer?

After we get home from a morning playgroup at Sara's, the children play, while I sit alone in the kitchen. Something nags me, a thought that escapes consciousness. I tap my pen against the tabletop, gaze out the window, and write some notes.

Could it be we have lived and died already, that this is the hell we live in fear of? Or are we merely approaching another Great Flood, another point in time when only a catastrophe can clean the world's slate? Has the world progressed to its logical, final conclusion as a result of wrong paths taken, a path leading to consummate evil, a place where the only solution is cataclysmic change or global annihilation?

The universe now seems to proceed in almost the reverse of what should be. Surely there are others who know the end is approaching, that things cannot proceed in this way. Has Sam been trying to guide me subtly to this realization? Is he one of a few prophets, or guides, who represent God in Her/His attempt to reverse reality? Or is Sam an aspect of God embodied in only a few people in this calamitous time? Has he been attempting to form me into an ally? Have we both, along with others, only now been allowed consciousness of our purpose on earth?

Maybe the world is not strictly reversed but only in part, a more chaotic disorder. Yesterday, Sam's and my sexual appearance, face-to-face, genitalia to genitalia, didn't form the Tao of wholeness, but instead was a reversal of one aspect. Not so simple. Within ourselves, the reversal of left brain controlling the right side of the body. Our eyes, the reversal on the retina reversed again by optic nerves.

What is within is without. We think of our bodies as containers when we are in fact like Einstein's concept of the universe, a torus, like a doughnut, the inner surface merely an extension of the outer. I laugh—people are rather like tubes. And what about the isomorphism between bodies, astral and human, between the universe and the eye?

Maybe meaning doesn't exist in the metaphysical, spiritual realm but instead imbues the concrete world. It lurks in invisibility because no one expects to find it there, like "The Purloined Letter," staring everyone in the face, but ignored. Car colors, the significance of their positions at Sam's yesterday. Green facing white, blue blocking yellow. My associations of people with colors: Jake, black with villainy, the red of blood, fire, the Devil. Sam, green, grassy earth, nature, life.

What is within appears in opposite form without, but still it is all one thing. Complementary colors are actually afterimages, functions of each other. People see redness because green is absorbed while red is reflected. It is yellow, the light, which is superordinate to black and white, to darkness and color, and which gives life to all.

Bea calls to arrange a babysitting exchange. I jot down *2:25, 9/24*, the time of her call, and *1:30–4:30, 9/28*, the babysitting date. I smile and think, *Is this, too, to be learned from rather than acted upon?*

I return to writing my notes. *What is the significance of the current time frame?* Yesterday, the autumnal equinox, 9/23, parallels the time of my birth at 9:23 p.m. Something significant about this point in time. Is it that there *is* no time? That time is folding in upon itself?

Are we nearing the juncture of all past, all future, where time will collapse in upon itself unless it is reordered? Or has time been running backward for all known history, and people's lives have proceeded in reverse while we mistakenly believed we were proceeding forward?

The calendar system is out of sync with reality, missing a month (thirteen lunar months vs. twelve calendar months, although sometimes the Hebrew calendar has thirteen), and plagued with slippage: *Sept* = 7, but September is the ninth month; *Oct* = 8, not 10; *Nov* = 9, not 11; *Dec* = 10, not 12.

Words are jumbled, in disarray. Everyone knows *dog* is *God* spelled backward, but also *Devil* = *lived*, and isn't this remarkable, the idea that the Devil is life in the past tense. How most of us live—creating our present as the past as we live in the future, planning, working toward, at the cost of the present.

I make coffee, sit at the kitchen table again, and draw diagrams of some of these new concepts.

"Mummy? What are you doing?" Jessie climbs onto my lap and reaches for my pen. "Can I draw too?"

I look at Jessie in surprise and quickly slip the notebook from under Jessie's hand and close it. "How about a snack while I change clothes?"

"An apple without the peeling, okay, Mom?" Jessie climbs off my lap and pulls the peeler out of the drawer.

"Hand that to me, please," I say.

Brandon runs into the kitchen, trips on the threshold, and lying on the floor, says, "Cottage cheese."

I shed the clothes I wore to the playgroup earlier in the day and put on purple underwear, a pink sweatshirt, my blue jeans.

Pink and blue outside, but purple underneath. Male and female outside, integrated underneath. I must be careful what I wear. I slip my bare feet into my white flip-flops. Pure white, reverence for what lies between my body and the earth.

I call Sam to arrange our meeting for next week but reach his answering machine. The red phone, the color of evil, connects with another machine. Appropriate. Their evil will cancel each other out—the words reversed twice will be conveyed in original form?

The children are quiet. I find them in the living room, sitting on the floor in the sunlight. They are carefully placing colored cars, green, white, yellow, blue, purple, on their toy plates. They are uncommonly intent on their design, and then I see the significance of the cars, their colors—their behavior is hooked into my unconscious. They line the cars up, and I see they have recreated the configuration of the cars at Sam's yesterday. Again the macrocosm in the concrete, the particular. I smile.

The cars become disordered again, and I note that the purple car, Jake's car, is lying upside down: an accident. He will not be home tonight after all. Brandon rams other cars into it. The cars lie in a jumbled pile. So gory. I reconsider, right the cars. No need for these deaths. I say it is time to clean up, and I place the cars on their plates once more, carefully preserving the balanced configuration. I am awed with the responsibility—what occurs within this house will be reflected in the world outside it.

Jake arrives home. He has been saved from accident after all. It is six thirty, and he asks, "What's on the menu?"

I say I'm not very hungry, have nothing planned—I've been too busy.

When I make no move to prepare a meal, he orders pizza. While Jake and the kids pick up the slices and eat it, I get a fork—pizza always burns the roof of my mouth. Why do I eat it? Jake, Italian. His food.

Jake starts to pour apple juice for the kids and himself, and I am annoyed. I insist, "The kids should have milk." Thinking, *mother's milk*, pure white, not apple juice, this defilement of the fruit. Why haven't I attended to the brand name before—*After the Fall*?

Jessie seems torn but agrees to milk, while Brandon chooses the apple juice. I am pleased about winning this half victory. I pour myself some milk, look at the pizza, and grimace. Red, like blood, something that will adulterate. I have not eaten that day, have forgotten to, but do not want to eat this.

When Jake frowns and says, "You're not eating," I force myself to take a bite or two and then say, "I'm not hungry," and push my plate away. I am not meant to eat this; it is the eating of his will. Something evil about it, the red of the Devil.

I smoke. I drink my milk, holy, purifying, a nurturing substance. I am like a newborn babe, so vital and open to the world.

I lie on my bed, smoking, and the kids bring me books to read to them. I am pleased that they ally themselves with me in a place where it is unusual for us to read together. I stub out my cigarette, and the three of us huddle together on our stomachs and start reading Maurice Sendak's *In the Night Kitchen*. I am enamored of the pictures, of their meanings, of the words.

Time is slowed, almost stops. I read one or two words very slowly but become lost in the profuse associations. So much richness on each page.

"Read, Mom, read!" the children prod me.

I stop again, smiling at the last lines in the book. The main character rejoices that he is both swimming in milk and it is also inside him, and then he prays for blessings on both the milk and himself. I read another book, by Marie Hall Ets, *Play with Me*. A young girl scares animals away by approaching them too eagerly—only when she sits still, silent, do they come play with her. So beautifully distracting, so difficult to read.

When the kids are asleep, I walk through my house following the light of my cigarette, watching it sketch circles in the dark air. I feel no fear. The darkness is warm. The cigarette like the moon, shining in the dark, Sam, the sun, resting while I, the moon, shine.

CHAPTER 19:

HERDING CHAOS

Saturday, 9/25, early morning. I go for a drive. I need cigarettes again. I drive toward the red brick building of the Arsenal, recalling my imagined suicide by driving into it, but instead turn left to buy cigarettes, my fuel, at the gas station. Back on Arsenal Street, I turn left at every green light, turning to what is left. Left is right, a transcendence of the dichotomy through reinterpretation.

As I drive, I think that Sam is resting now, staying home to leave, while I provide the protective encircling of my home. Perhaps the yellow car at Sam's is metaphorical? Perhaps our journey will be some other kind altogether? A form of virginity, another form of Virginia? I, too, am meant to stay home, to reflect him. In staying, I will leave. I must stay with the children.

Sam returns my call from yesterday afternoon. A day later, I think. He says that if we meet on Tuesday, it will have to be at 7:30 a.m., but if we meet on Wednesday, we must meet earlier, at 7:00 a.m. He asks whether I understand, implying some underlying meaning to this discrepancy: If we meet earlier, it will be later; if later, earlier. He says to find out what is convenient for Jake's schedule (he must watch the kids), and to call him back by 11:20, because he is going out. His voice sounds dusty, husky, and broken by pauses, as if it is a strain talking though this instrument, this red phone.

Does the phone transform voices through the medium of its evil? Was it really Sam who called, or could it have been Joy, disguised, attempting to thwart our meeting? What did he mean about leaving? He is vacating? Fasting? Joy will be in control?

How am I to interpret his signs? When is this great meeting to take place really? What is the vortex at which time will fold together? Did he literally mean Tuesday or Wednesday, or are they only clues I am to understand? Today, the Jewish Sabbath; tomorrow, Sunday, the Christian Sabbath. There has been a slippage so the two Sabbaths do not coincide. Are we to meet Sun-day? Or Wednesday, Weds-day? It's all too confusing. Oh, God, what if I don't figure out what he means in time? I run to the drawer and pull out my notebook.

If clock time and calendar time are distorted, maybe they should be read in reverse. Or if time is running backward, perhaps our meeting will fold back into 1981, when Sam and I first met. I cannot figure it out! But I breathe a sigh of relief—maybe I am not meant to, but instead, to follow my intuition.

Sam had suggested asking Jake—maybe he is saying to let Jake have his way, to follow his will, and in complying, I will subordinate it to my own. Yes. I call to Jake, who is in the living room with the kids, and he confirms what I have suspected—Wednesday is best. It fits—wedding day.

I call Sam, but Joy answers, even though I called within the specified time. Has she discovered our planned meeting? Is she in league with Jake? I feel Sam is there, in the background, unable to come to the phone in Joy's presence. Both Sam and I are to allow ourselves to be subject to this evil to overcome it. Or is it really Sam, able to speak to me only by transforming his voice so the message can be given through two reversals? That of the instrument of the Devil, the red phone, and that of a changed voice?

I explain nonchalantly to "Joy" that Sam has asked me to return his call. She says he'll call back in a few minutes. When the phone rings, I ask Jake to answer it, to tell Sam I will meet with him on Wednesday. In this way, the message will be clarified through two reversals, the evil of the phone and that of Jake. Jake appears to be talking to Sam, but I cannot be sure, perhaps it is Joy, their pretense.

Jake asks whether everything will be okay if he takes Jessie to the supermarket. Why does he ask? I nonchalantly say Brandon will probably nap while they are gone, and I will too—I didn't sleep very well last night.

I fool him. Once he's gone, I have things to do. Perhaps now Sam will come for me. Maybe he'll come to my door as long as I stay home. I must prepare for him.

I step into the kids' room. Brandon naps quietly, thumb in mouth, hugging his white teddy, his yellow blankie scrunched tightly in his hand. His innocence touches me. Is he an infant Sam who coexists with his adult form through some overlapping in time? Or is Brandon instead a tiny Brian? Or a reconstituted me? While rebellious Jessie is a small Brian, the personalities and the sexes reversed in this current manifestation? A test: Can I make it end differently? I must, I must.

Oh, my God, the cloth dolls, limbs poking every which way from the toy shelves. Mangled. Sam must not see these. I turn the dolls so they face the back of the shelves and cover them with stuffed animals. The animal faces, too, I turn inward—none must see. Simultaneously, the cloth dolls in the world will be concealed—as I prepare my home, so the world will be prepared.

But what of the Strawberry Shortcake lunch box atop the refrigerator? Are even pictures of cloth dolls taboo? I walk to the refrigerator, rust-colored, the color of Sam's hair, and take down the lunch box sitting atop it, shove it into a lower cabinet, and then, on second thought, remove it so I can neutralize the thermos inside that so often contains apple juice. I pour milk into it, then place it on the counter. I eye the radio—music, the essence of Sam—and turn it on, angling it toward the lunch box, a further neutralization. I cut off the toaster, the evil heat, by placing the protective blender before it, its blades intervening between the lunch box and the instrument of heat.

Everything is so disordered! Why haven't I seen the illogic of the world, of the things in this house, before? How the placement of household items defies the natural order, has been an attempted cancellation of what is natural, a product of an evil influence I have not even observed consciously.

The potatoes, roots from under the earth, atop the refrigerator should be at ground level, away from light. Same with the onions. I open the refrigerator door. Mind-boggling! I separate the apple juice from the milk. Milk on the top shelf. Eggs belong there too. Separate the red of the ketchup, representing blood, evil, from the other items. Apples grow above ground, so should be on the top shelf, not in the drawer, but they too are red, so there needs to be a separating influence. I move the meat away from the milk, the red from the purity, the Jewish separation of milk and meat. I peek into the freezer. The chocolate ice cream sits atop the vanilla ice cream; evil subjugates good, so I reverse them and place the vanilla upside down atop the chocolate, creating the Tao. I have done what I can, yet there are too many contaminating categories to know whether my reordering is correct. I give up, leaving some food on the counters.

But what of the toys? Their placement is totally illogical—toy cars and trucks in the living room and riding toys everywhere. I pile them near the doorway—they belong in the garage. In the bedroom, I find the toy dishes, which should be in the dining room. I remove them from the shelves, piling them atop the clothes, freshly laundered days ago, still awaiting folding. Finally I see the reordering is an impossible task—and anyway, the disorder is a form of order—distracting me from my ordained task.

So stuffy in the house. Brandon sleeps, too long. I sit next to him, but cannot see him breathe—is he dying? Already dead?

I shake him lightly. His eyelids flutter, and he moans that his head hurts. I think, yes, my head hurt, too, when all this started—some alteration is being made in his mind, as in mine, so that he too will join me in this newly disclosed reality. It is Brandon and I who will be the eyes, responsible for reversing this evil that only we have been designated to see. Because others can't see it, I cannot even speak of it.

Or has the whole world sifted down into a reverse reality, like the sand in an hourglass, into a hell parallel to our former heaven? It is a conjunction of realities, both heaven and hell, and which reality will prevail depends on me and others. A volleying for control that must happen silently, without acknowledgment on anyone's part that there is this game at all. All pretend that life proceeds as usual, a rule of this most serious of games.

I walk down the street with Brandon, my white flip-flops a protective membrane between me and the cement, this man-made chain atop the earth.

Brandon, a child of wisdom, leads me. He stops at the playground, asks to swing. I push him.

When I ask where else he would like to go, he leads me farther from our house. Have I constrained him to a world too small?

As we approach a basketball court, he points and says, "baseball," and then pointing to a baseball diamond, he says, "basketball." Are we each wandering in our own separate reality?

After crossing an open field, we come to Mount Auburn Street, and Brandon wishes to cross. I lift him into my arms. The cars race past, cutting space in two with their hard, hot metal. Will they never stop?

After waiting, waiting, waiting, we cross, and I set him down. He bends down, picks up a stone, and says, "popcorn," and I see again that reality has been disordered. Or we hold hands at the juncture of two realities.

Brandon leads me up a side street as if to show me something. An older boy, maybe six, approaches us on his tricycle, and his younger sister, maybe four, runs after him. Both have auburn-colored hair. They stop, silently watching Brandon and me, so we stop too. The kids turn, returning up the hill and around the corner.

We follow, finding them in a yard, as if waiting for us. A Holly Hobbie doll sits near the swing set, and hanging in the windows of this white house are my curtains, white with orange stripes. Is this Sam's and my home in an alternative reality? These, our children? Does he wait inside for me to recognize my true home? All the signs: a reality in which cloth dolls are without threat; a white house, a pure home, the reverse of my brown one; the children with his hair.

The children reverse my children, the boy two years older than the girl. Sam and I in another aspect? Or a reversal of my own childhood, Brian now older than me? The boy says his sister's birthday is Christmas Day. I wonder if the significant historical event to occur will be a woman's emergence, this little girl, as the new Christ, the savior.

Must I do something now to activate this reality, make it ascendant? I study the curtains. Does Sam silently watch there in the dark? The reverse of my dream in which I stand in the darkness outside, while he, in the light, invites me in. And yet, where is the invitation?

As we climb the hill to our own house, I see a group of people gathered there, our neighbors.

I ask Jake, "Why are there so many people here? Did something happen?"

"I was worried. We came home and there wasn't a note, and you weren't at the playground, so I asked the neighbors if they'd seen you."

A bit dumbfounded, I shake my head. "We just went for a walk." I lift Brandon into my arms and head inside.

Later. It is dark. A horn honks. Is it Sam coming for me?

I walk outside, hear a dog bark, and see a car to my right, lights on, honking, in front of the house next door. As I walk toward it, it backs up the hill. I stop, walk backward, and it approaches. Again, I approach and it backs up. This is not the place we will meet.

I turn and walk down the street, carefully sidestepping the light from the streetlamps, weaving around them, moving in darkness, encircling Sam in this way, while he works in the light.

I come to the playground. Perhaps we will meet in a metaphorical environment, as pure as children who in their wisdom can change the world. Yet we must meet backward, upside down, to create the Tao.

I climb the slide, backward, my back to the steps, and wait, but he does not come. Trial and error to discover the correct place. I slide down backward, then try the blue swing, but I am too big in this little world, and I laugh.

I eye the stationary stagecoach—of course!—those fantasy monkey bars, where we will stay to leave, sit immobile to move. But still he doesn't appear.

I walk down the middle of a side street, so happy I can walk in the dark. I have been unnecessarily afraid of it—there is warmth and love in this darkness, no need to fear—his love encloses me. I weave my way around the lights and finally return home. I must always return home.

I am surprised to find Donna there. An odd time—late for her to come by. Has she been drawn to me? Is she an unknowing disciple in Sam's and my venture? Her eyes are bloodshot, perhaps tired from her efforts.

"Why are you here?" I ask her, as we sit down on the sofa.

"I was just wondering how you're doing, and—"

Jake interrupts, "I asked her to watch the kids so I could go find you."

"I was just out for a walk. I needed some fresh air," I say, as Brandon crawls onto the sofa and squeezes between us.

"But you never walk alone in the dark," Jake insists.

"Well, I do now. I'm a woman taking back the night." I smile at Donna, who attends Women Take Back the Night rallies.

I hear a sound outside and jump up to open the shades. I must be able to see. I cannot speak of the transformation of the world to Donna, to anyone. So difficult, bearing this burden of silence, but the world is not ready to hear. A car horn honks repeatedly, beckoning me, and, as my eyes dart to the window, Donna in turn eyes me suspiciously.

When she finally leaves, I sit on the porch steps and smoke, then carry my butts to a pothole in the center of the street, not to adulterate the earth, the grass. Appropriate to place the ashes on the asphalt, the man-made chains binding the earth, a sacrificial offering, a ritualistic cleansing through applying the dead ash to the technology of death. Ashes to ashes.

Jake joins me on the porch, sits next to me, a sign I am to go in. If he's out, I must be inside. I counter his actions. When he reenters the house, I again leave. No room for both of us.

He calls to me through the screen door. "Aren't you coming to bed?"

I decide I am to squelch his act by complying, opposing his expectation that I will not comply. So I return.

I lie in bed, smoking, and in the basement window of the house next door, I see an answering flame. Is it merely a reflection? I wave my cigarette to see. It is not. It's a tiny light like my own. Sam is there? I extend my hand to him, whispering, "Please come to me."

I hear the wind, the rustle of the grass, and yes, he is below my window. He walks around this house, encircling me, protecting me, just as I have encircled him in my journeying.

I carefully crawl out of bed, down on my hands and knees, and avoiding the light, peer out. He is just below me to my right. But I am not meant to see him there—if I look, he will disappear. What must be done must occur beneath observation.

I return to bed but soon hear a car honking. I leave the house, but it is quiet outside, the car gone, so I return, settle into the rocker, smoke, turn on the music quietly. Maybe Sam is conveying messages to me through lyrics. "Every Breath You Take," a song by The Police, is one of several with messages to me—the music slows just as time slows; the songs continue far past their normal length, and certain refrains are played over and over, to ensure I will hear them.

Sam says, via Neil Diamond, to switch on my "Heartlight," and I turn on the ceiling light. But is it this light he means? My refrigerator dream, food flying when the door opens, the light shining out, the power of it.

I go to the refrigerator, hold the door open, let this heartlight shine out, and, at the same time, turn on the radio in the pantry, so I can continue to follow his messages. Back to The Police . . . Sam says he'll be watching me . . . I crouch between the open refrigerator door and the window, trying to see where he is. In the house behind rather than in front, where I see a light? While I sit in darkness, Taoist opposition.

I decide to check the houses next door to ours. To our left is another brown shingle, my house's twin, and in the window of the bedroom is a flowering plant that was not there before, a sign to me that he is there, love is there, something flourishing. I am not alone; he watches, protects me.

From another window, I see lights in the kitchen of the house to my right and once again there are new additions—hanging plants. Someone moves about in that kitchen, someone with gray hair. I am viewing an alternative future, something that might happen—my choice. It is our home, Sam's and mine, in the distant future. We have grown old together.

Must I go there to activate this future? Are the plants the invitation, the signal? I step outside, walk to the front of the neighboring house. Am I to enter this house—green, Sam's color?

But with no obvious invitation, I turn, walk to the brown house. Which house? How am I to know? Why such an obscure puzzle?

Back inside, I peer out the window and watch the sunrise, thinking now I may rest, finally. But an oddity strikes me—there are no cars on the street. Even our landlord has been influenced to do the bizarre, his car pulled onto the grass of the yard. It is as if my dream of the future has been externalized, the one in which there are no cars on the street and I am searching for Sam. The neighbors, too, have been impelled to park elsewhere, not knowing why, not even questioning, unconscious pawns of my power, of Sam's power.

CHAPTER 20:

GARDEN OF EDEN OR THE DEVIL'S FIRST SUPPER

Sunday morning, 9/26: The whole family is outside again. Jake has rolled my Bug to the bottom of the driveway and is changing the oil, putting the discarded oil in an empty milk carton, replacing the nourishing milk with black oil, evil blighting the innocent container. I watch as he dumps it over the fence into the neighbor's yard.

Midmorning, the children have not eaten, so I take them inside.

"We want apple juice!" Jessie says.

Brandon joins in, "Apple juice!" And then starts thumb-sucking again.

"You have to drink milk." I pour milk into their glasses, despite their protests.

"Can we have eggs?" Jessie asks, although they never want eggs, and then clarifies, "Boiled eggs."

Brandon pulls his thumb out, and says, "Eggs!" As if it were Easter.

I must cooperate but somehow forestall this eating of eggs. I have said to Sam, "I feel like an egg, so fragile." The cosmic egg. I put a pot of water on over a low flame, lower the eggs into tepid water, and pretend to cook them. They are like the universe, the yellow yolk floating in its transparent albumen, the yellow center enclosed by its surroundings, feeding each other, dependent on each other, within this delicate shell. What happens in the microcosm, electrons orbiting atomic nuclei, happens in the macrocosm, planets orbiting the sun, so why not in the mediocosm, in everyday reality? What happens at one level, happens at another.

But what if the eggs should crack?! Maybe if the eggs crack, the whole universe will explode in a cosmic bang, a gunshot to the temple of the universe, and the whole world will disintegrate! Their interiors must not harden, the center must remain fluid, in some balance between hard and formless runniness—my seemingly mundane task is actually nothing less than determining the appropriate consistency of the entire universe. I must be very, very, very careful how I cook these eggs—maybe just warm them. I should aim for the warmth of the sun, reflected in and out, in the center of the delicate egg and in the water, the fluidity that surrounds it.

Jessie asks, "When are the eggs gonna be done, Mumma?"

I smile and use Sam's phrase, "There is time."

Jake enters, peeks into the pot, and notices the low flame. "They'll never get cooked that way." He turns up the heat full blast.

The uncontrolled heat of hell is what he would apply to the cosmic egg! As soon as he steps away, I turn down the flame. The eggs may not cook! I am overwhelmed with my task, so delicate, and yet so far, no cracks in the shells.

Jake comes over. "The eggs must be done by now."

"I think they're just right," I say.

He cracks one open.

I cringe and quietly moan, "Noooo"—but it is too late!

"Why, these eggs aren't even cooked!" he says with disgust, before dumping them into the disposal.

I am tense with worry, but all is okay—the universe continues, and the eggs have not been eaten.

The kids cry for their eggs, and I say, "You shouldn't be eating eggs anyway."

But Jake is determined, cracks some open and fries them in oil, and I am disgusted. When he turns to set the table, I turn the heat off under the eggs.

Jake accuses me, "Now you're denying the kids food?"

"Too many eggs aren't good for them—you say that yourself all the time."

The eggs are fried, but maybe it's okay as long as they are not consumed. After Jake places the plates on the table and turns again, I casually drop ashes from my cigarette onto the eggs—they will not be eaten!

Jake is furious and dumps the fried eggs in the disposal.

"It was an accident," I say, even though I know he won't believe it.

He serves the kids Cheerios, little O's again, the tiny doughnuts of the universe. He is determined to feed them this universe, but it's okay—Cheerios, the dead and baked grain, removed enough from life, so eating them will have no important impact.

Jake asks when I have last eaten, and I say, "I'm not hungry."

The milk nourishes, and I am energized with smoke. Energy surges through my veins. I am empowered, do not need food, have no needs, will not eat of this life. As I fast, so does Sam, emptying his being of impurity. Today Yom Kippur begins—of course, he does not eat.

Jake's mother, Teri, calls. We are coming to the family picnic, aren't we? No need to worry about bringing food. She will provide enough food for everyone, fried chicken and some Italian dishes.

Yes, I think, Teri would very much like us to eat the "food," the desecrated chicken, dead flesh, the diabolical sauces. I can picture the "family" sitting behind a long table—the Devil's family. Why haven't I seen it before? But they are only now attempting to arise, and today is the critical day, the Last Supper in reverse, the Devil presiding instead of Jesus, ready to ascend into power. It will be a ritual meal, eating flesh, drinking blood in the guise of those red, spicy sauces.

But we've also been invited to go apple picking with my friends Donna, Sara, and Bea and their families. The calendar reads "apple picking or family picnic," picking or picnic: the fall from grace in the garden, picking the apples, the apples of knowledge of good and evil, or the Devil's First Supper, the arise of the Devil. My friends or his family, what am I meant to do? Stay to leave, comply to defy. I decide it is Jake's choice. My role is to follow him and counteract him in some way. He wants to go to the picnic, so I agree.

I try to delay by insisting the kids must be bathed—they are dirty, unwashed, must be cleansed, for *these my children* are to be offered up to His family. As I'm dressing them, Jake appears, wearing his red shirt with black stripes, the perfect representation, the red fires of hell behind bars. I dress the children in white and blue, Jessie in a white-and-blue striped top like my own, to counteract the red and black of Jake. Jessie says, "Mummy and me are twins," and I am glad we are allied in this way.

As we gather our things, I hear the news on the radio: There is a moose on the loose, wandering along the highways of New Hampshire, just avoiding cars—it must be Sam transformed; he is up north inscribing an arc in his travels to reflect my movement south to Canton, as if we are on opposing ends of a swinging pendulum. He compensates, counteracts my journey, this weighty event we are about to attend.

Jake is driving down Route 128, encircling Boston, heading south to Canton, an anagram for *Cannot*, the perfect name for hell, half the word reversed and folded in upon itself, a form of masturbation. But I am in control. I wave my cigarette as if sketching in the air, influencing where he drives, and just barely saving us, repeatedly. Jake pretends not to notice.

We exit onto a side street, Pleasant Road, passing a cemetery—it is dead here, the buried dead. But we are lost, lost in Cannot, and it seems ordained—an effect of the confusion here, the chaos. Jake stops, asks directions. Someone says, "You can't miss the park—you'll see a large white house," but when we arrive, the house is purple. It is a different park, situated in hell, in a reverse reality. Perhaps the transformation coincided with the coming of this evil family, which disorders, defiles.

On the open field facing us, a group of young men, each with carrot-red hair, are playing football. They stop their game just as Jake pulls our car to a stop, and these guardians of hell whisper to each other, then wander over to where we are parked, watching, watching. I stare at them, squint my eyes with all the power I can collect, and will them to stay away. I shiver—it is so cold here.

I think Jake's family is not here, but he points them out atop a long hill, clustered around tables aligned under a series of trees, as if even though it is dark, cloudy, they require this added protection from the sun since it is antithetical to their beings. As we walk slowly up the hill, I am filled with a sense of portent—the trees above the family are wild with the wind. So cold and dark here. I must follow Jake, but how can I turn back time and avert this catastrophic moment that threatens all mankind?

Jake's mother greets us with chicken, wants us to *take, eat, in remembrance of . . .*

I say, "I'm not hungry."

I do not let the children eat, but instead gather them to me, and say, "I'm leaving. It's too cold here—the children have no jackets, no protection."

I rush them down the hill, avoiding disaster, the Event, and Jake comes running after us.

In the car, he turns to me and says, "What the hell? If you didn't want to come, you could have said so."

"Who knew it would be so cold here?"

Jake is again huddled over the wheel—can he feel he is not in control? The radio is on, and I hear that the moose in New Hampshire is still wandering around, crazed, and hunting parties are trying to capture it. I am anxious to get home, so Sam, who has assumed the guise of the moose, can finally rest.

At home in Watertown, it is warm again. It was cold only in Canton. Since I did not eat the Devil's food in Canton, under the watchful eyes of those carrot-heads, Jake decides to make a carrot cake—an abomination of ingredients, degraded from their natural forms. Carrot cake, his preferred birthday cake—he is determined he shall be born today, that the Devil shall gain ascendance.

I protest. "But you don't know how to bake it, and we don't have all the ingredients."

"We do," he insists, as he gathers together the instruments of this destructive construction: the knives, the blades, the peelers, the food processor, that which cuts, separates, works in the aid of disintegration.

He gives the children peelers for the carrots, and he too is peeling. It is as if he wants the children to be cut, hurt.

"They're too young!" I say as I watch their little hands and his larger ones flying together over the sink, hands, knives, cutting, flying, in careless waves. Finally, I say, "I'll peel the carrots." Anything, anything, to save the children.

I am peeling the carrots and wondering, *Do the carrots feel their skin torn away from their interiors? Could they have some consciousness of pain but be unable to signal it?* But I make this sacrifice for the children—the peeling is inevitable.

But I must also observe, for Jake is chopping the nuts with a butcher knife, and the children are standing on chairs, staggering on their still-wobbly legs, and he is blind to it, cannot visualize them falling onto the cutting board, their fingers severed. I find that just as a child is about to fall, I can correct for his or her balance by turning in the opposing direction, as the children's movements seem to be a function of Jake's and mine. And so, as Jake turns and Brandon begins to fall, stumbling, his foot stepping off the edge of the chair, I turn in a direction opposed to Jake's, before the act occurs, as if I can turn back time, forestall the inevitable, act in the interstices between one moment and the last. Turn back time, I have to turn back time.

Eventually the carrots are done, sitting on the counter, quietly awaiting their terrible fate, and I cannot intervene—I am to passively observe, intervening only by my movement, invisibly correcting, or by announcing what is happening, not telling him what to do, since Jake must experience the consequences of his own actions: Brandon is falling, the eggs are too close to the edge of the table, etc. I am terrified of accidents yet must not interfere.

The kitchen is altered with the careless flurry of Jake's activity—he is at the center generating chaos. There are carrot shreds on the walls, on the floor, egg dripping from the table, brown sugar underfoot, eggshells littering the sink, and flour spilled. The kids are covered in flour, brown sugar stuck to their shirts in little sandy globs. It is perfect evidence of the disorder, the filth, the chaos that ascends when Jake is given sway.

I cannot interfere with the making of the cake, but can help with the cleanup. I gather together the remnants of this unholy effort, placing it all in the sink, eggshells, carrot shreds, scattered flour, sugar, nuts, until the disposal is so overfilled that the sink is clogged and looks like a regurgitation, as if the earth will not accept this defilement. But then the disposal painfully does accept this Devil's vomit with a great extended belch; it passes down its throat to its belly. It is Sam accepting all this, swallowing it to contain the evil. I wonder how he manages, how he can be capable of accepting, transforming, so much evil. I watch, reverently.

Finally, the cake is in the red Bundt pan and in the oven. The timer must be set, and it must be set twice, the cake requiring more than an hour. It is critical for me to time this right, but then I see the clocks all display different times, and I panic. Why haven't I noticed this before? Is this Jake's attempt to confuse my concept of time, to prevent what must be done at the critical point? And does it relate to the baking of the cake? When it's done, will the world be forever altered?

I run from room to room, the kitchen clock, the stove clock, the bedroom clocks, the living room clock, my watch—I must coordinate them all. But how am I to know the critical moment?

Back in the kitchen, I watch with dread as the cake bakes—it is a countdown. Something awful will happen when the buzzer goes off, something irrevocably horrendous. The universal bang? *Bang, bang*, we're all dead. I watch the kitchen clock, see it slow, and then, with all my powers of concentration, I make the clock turn backward. It is just barely perceptible, but I must make time flow backward, must give Sam the time he needs. *That* is my critical function. Today is the day, at five o'clock, when the cake is to be done, the beginning of Yom Kippur, and Jake is trying to make it Easter with the carrots, the eggs, fighting to maintain the old order, the separation of Jew and Christian. Of Sam and me?

Finally, finally, the cake is done. I have done something right. There are no apparent consequences; I have foiled him. Jake offers the cake to the kids and me, further defiling it with scoops of ice cream. I accept a piece but do not eat—say I am not hungry after all. The kids listen, and they eat only a few bites, do not consume what Jake has created, will not be so easily influenced.

It is Yom Kippur, and perhaps Sam is awaiting me, fasting in some empty room, my rightful home. I leave the house, walk down the middle of the street—I must not harm the earth with my weight, the depressions of my feet. I create crosses with my footsteps, purifying the streets, rendering them harmless.

There is so much construction in the neighborhood, houses being restored, a turning inside out of my own mind, reflecting the construction within. The workers altering the houses are unaware of their roles, of being actors in my play. Now, as I watch them, I think they are aware, always have been, have been waiting for me to become aware of my own role—all the world has been preparing me; they are all superb actors, acting as though they would continue in their activities even if I were not observing—so nonchalant, so realistic. I catch them looking at me and pretending I am insignificant to their lives.

I study the houses, trying to divine in which one Sam waits. It must be some reverse of my own home. Around the block, I find another brown shingle, a mirror image of our house. It is numberless, nameless; perhaps it is my home. Someone is working in the upstairs room—I see movement there. An empty house being constructed—for me? Sam inside, waiting for me to recognize my own home? He must stay hidden until I enter, cannot give me clues. Yet I will not act without invitation, unlike Brian, following that dog into a house uninvited. But what will constitute that invitation if we must act in silence?

As I return home, I see a carload of people unloading picnic items and beer. Loud and boisterous, they emerge onto the second-floor porch of the house directly across the street, as if they are to perform a play for me, and is that Sam up there? The auburn hair, but it is difficult to tell from where I stand. Where are the women who live there? It is bizarre, the two women not among the players, as if these strangers have taken over the apartment.

I start walking around the block again, to enclose it twice, once in each direction, but as I proceed, the loud talk from the porch ceases. I am making an error, their silence tells me. So I start to walk in the other direction and again the noise ceases. I am the actor, they the audience—I perform to their responses. Am I to go home again? I start toward my door, and again they quiet. I search their remote faces and then feel totally frustrated. I return to the center of the street, facing them. I wave the gold key in my hand and yell, "What is it you want me to do?!"

As they watch, I let my head drop back and mimic swallowing the key like a fish, and then I lift my leg and mimic incorporating it vaginally, and they are silent. Under my breath, I say, "Fuck you," and go to my door. As I open it, I can hear them talking. When I turn, they stop, and I frown at them. Whose side are they on? I slam the door.

Donna calls. "How was the picnic?"

I say, "It was too cold. We didn't stay."

Donna tells me of the apple picking, how they drove to the orchard but instead found themselves at the strawberry patch where we had picked strawberries earlier this year.

I smile. It is time folding, spring and fall, strawberries and apples. They have been drawn to that particular place, drawn by Sam's and my wills to that strawberry patch, the living expression of Sam's phobia, the representative in reality of a Strawberry Shortcake cloth doll. I am amused, amazed by the "coincidence."

Although I am silent, Donna continues, telling of an unusual sight they have seen. Walking along the country road was a woman leading a pregnant donkey.

I think it is a reversal of history, the replacement of Christ riding the donkey on Palm Sunday, like the Zen "riding the bull," only in this case it is a progression, the spirit contained in the donkey, not atop it, and a woman leads it, rather than a man riding it. Sam has worked this, or Sam and I together, our psyches creating in reality the concrete evidence of our spiritual union. The woman represents me, Sam the donkey. Or the donkey, the mother, is me, and Sam is transformed into a woman—it is all an externalization of inner reality to outer. A transformation in the world. The donkey encircles the space where Sam and I will unite, just as the moose on the loose does in New Hampshire.

Sam has been very busy, manifesting himself in the moose too. He must be exhausted, but we cannot sleep. The world depends on it. I would like to explain all of this to Donna, but it would be too much of a stretch, too far beyond Donna's experience for her to grasp, so I merely say "Hmm" or "Interesting" as Donna talks on until finally I say goodbye.

It is later, twilight, and the kids are fighting, torn between Jake and me, so I go outside. I draw a cross in front of my house through my walking and then hear the screams inside. It is hell in there; the windows glow red. As I walk, I notice white paint spattered on the driveway and front sidewalk—but is it actually paint? The landlord painted the trim this past summer, but it was not this profuse. It is as if semen has fallen on the house in the guise of paint, Jake's or the Devil's, if Jake is but a disciple. I encircle the house, trying to contain the evil, and realize I have made the female symbol, the invisible cross now attached to the circle I made.

I sit on the front steps, rest. Two boys whiz by on a bicycle, engaging in anal sex as they ride—raw sexuality, exposed, so obviously hell here, the boys showing no compunction about their public display.

Jake pokes his head out the door, urges me to bed, says I have not been sleeping enough. I go inside, must comply. He asks if I am going to undress, and I say I'm too tired, but really I must be prepared. I lie in bed, listen to his hollow sighs, peer out the window, listening to the distant noises of cars, trucks, of the world, and then the sound of a million voices, the dead crying, a morbid symphony, crying for release from the roads that enchain them, locking them into death. It is an appeal, *Please help, free us*, and I arise.

But what must I do? Maybe I am wrong to think what must be done must be accomplished outside my house. Perhaps it is something I must do here inside. I turn on the living room lights, open the shade. For us to meet, to open the metaphorical door, is there something I must do physically? Maybe arrange my physical body in a certain way? Stand on my head? Somersault (a rolling "O" of oneness, the "all")? My gymnastics achieving nothing, I eventually give up.

I am not understanding something. Is it this? That he, the sun, cannot meet me at night? The night is my realm, I, the moon. And what happens if the sun and the moon meet? Universal light, but signaling the end of the universe. Is this what I am meant to know? That we must always work together but may never meet after all?

CHAPTER 21:

FIGHTING FIRE WITH FIRE

Monday, 9/27. Jessie misses the carpool when I attempt to keep her home from school, but she insists on going, so Jake says he'll drive her to nursery school and will take Brandon with him. I ask him to buy me cigarettes while he's out—he can supply me with that which is necessary because of his evil.

In my bedroom, I study my clothes. My jeans, usually tight, sag from my frame—I smile at the success of my "vacation," the loss of emotional weight. I feel vital, my blood surging, red and blue blood, purple me.

Jake returns with my cigarettes, and I smoke and smoke. I must always have one lit—this little flame must persist, my only protection.

I leave the house, circle it clockwise, and stop to absorb the sun—it feels like arms enclosing me. Why haven't I felt this love before? I come to the stone in the middle of our backyard. The flat stone is so unusual, alone there. Like Stonehenge, perhaps it is an altar, marking a spot significant to space and time. I am meant to stand on it. I raise my arms to the sun, turn slowly in the tiny space, feet to the stone, which reaches down to the very center of the earth; I am to bleed on this stone, and I will my blood to flow from me, the Great Mother.

I can feel my love radiating outward to embrace the earth—my love, Sam's love, holding the world together. We are strong, will transcend and transform the world with this love that can contain all, that will prevail. I stand on my tiptoes, think I may ascend into the sky, float above and meet him there, our spirits rising above and enclosing the universe.

Later, Jake stands in the driveway and tells me he wants to adjust the timing on my car. I see him slip something into his back pocket—maybe spark plugs? I smile—I am going nowhere anyway. As I proceed up the driveway, I see there are leafy branches strewn between the two cars, and I think of Sam's yellow car also sitting at the end of his driveway, Joy's car blocking the way. How can Jake and Joy believe this will stop us?

The large branches look like palm fronds. I check to see whether nearby bushes have recently been trimmed, but they have not. And the foliage differs, and it has not been windy enough to break such large branches and blow them here. Sam must have come in the night, sanctified the separation, strewing the palms. Palms in September, a rotation of the calendar, Palm Sunday. A reversal of metaphorical time, yesterday the analog of Easter, the beginning of Yom Kippur; today, the analog of Palm Sunday. Time is unwinding backward as planned.

I take Brandon inside to drink milk together, purify ourselves, and then peruse the newspaper. I read an account of the moose in New Hampshire, finally struck by a car and then shot—how could they do that to the moose? Nature trying to assert itself into civilization and then murdered, as if murder were civilized. Is Sam okay? Surely he escaped in time, removed the spiritual extension of himself before the gunshot.

Brandon turns on the television, and I sit with him and simply cannot, cannot, believe my eyes. A man lies in a hospital bed, blood flowing from bandages around his head, blood on his cheeks, rolling into the crevices around his mouth, into his eyes. He is speaking to someone with nonchalance, while Brandon watches, sees this gore, and sucks his thumb, showing no reaction—it is a travesty. I turn the channel.

On public television, a jester enters a restaurant and speaks to a waiter in French. The waiter comes and goes. The jester refuses the food, sends it back. The jester looks at me and repeats certain words—a message. Then the clip runs in reverse until the jester is at the door again. This time he speaks in English, the same conflict occurs, and still he does not eat the food. It is all presented too carefully, the words so carefully enunciated, the jester peering at me, laughing. Is this something I am to understand? He returns to the table twice, and still he does not eat. Or is it a mockery—a jester, laughing in my face—a crude representation of my communication with Sam, something to confuse me? I jump up and turn off the TV, and Brandon cries. He wants the TV on.

Jake comes in, turns it back on, serving this abomination up to his son. When Jake leaves, I turn the TV sound off, and turn the stereo on instead, but Brandon turns the volume up again. I yield. Maybe it is only hell inside this house? I go out onto the porch, peer through the living room window at the TV—maybe it will appear normal from outside?

Jake walks into the living room and stops short when he sees me looking through the window. He motions for me to come in, then steps onto the porch and says Bea is on the phone.

I take the red phone, the transformer of voices, and hold it to my ear. I am silent, the sound of one hand clapping, that which has no name, and after a moment Bea speaks, but I am sure it is Sam's voice in disguise.

"Linda? Linda? Are you there? I just want you to know that no matter what you're going through, I'll always be your friend."

I manage an "Uh-hmm."

Bea/Sam says goodbye, meaning I am to stay here, constrain the evil to this house, make sure it does not spread, try to transform it, keep it within and alter it. The conflict is within these confines—it is here it will happen. I must not leave home, must drive the evil out.

Jessie returns home from nursery school via the carpool. I am greatly relieved when she says she is all right. I send Jake out for more cigarettes, and at last he is gone.

He brings me two cartons, not the three packs I requested. Is he implying it will be a long siege? That I will have to smoke all of these before it is accomplished? I am so tired of the endless smoke I must blow for protection.

He smiles at me as he hands me the cartons, and says, "You seem to have smoked five packs since yesterday—aren't you overdoing it?"

"You're making me! You're the one buying all the cigarettes—I don't even want to smoke."

I grab the cartons, run out the front door, deposit them in the trash, and toss my lighter in after them, but then pull out my lighter—it can be my protective light. I return through the back door, only to find Jake gone, retrieving the cigarettes. When he brings them in, I take them and run out the back door. If I go out the opposite door, maybe the cigarettes will stay put in the trash. But Jake goes out the front door and pulls them out yet again.

When he returns, I insist, "I don't want any cigarettes in this house."

He shoves them in a paper bag and hides them. Later, I find them outside the back door, waiting for me, and decide I must smoke after all, endlessly, until this is all over—it is my only protection. I bring them in again.

Now it is countdown time to some moment of irreparable destruction. It is Jake and me, one-to-one—I must not let him out of my sight. I follow him relentlessly, revolving around him, speaking nonstop, narrating what is happening around him, "The kids are falling off their chairs, the water is boiling, the refrigerator door is open," trying to extinguish his light with my own.

He backs away—I am powerful with my smoke. I blow it in his eyes, in his ears, in his face, surround him. When he does one thing, I counteract him by doing the opposite. He tries to leave the room, but I turn in the opposite direction, and always he comes back. I control him. He submits.

Sam calls. I overhear Jake say, "She needs to see you." I am pleased the enemy has arranged our meeting. Now that Jake is speaking to him, Sam is in control—finally I may rest.

I lie down on our bed, shut my eyes, but still must convey to Sam the hell that exists here, but indirectly, and so I moan, hoping he will hear. I cannot keep my eyes shut, so I jump up and approach Jake. I cannot speak directly to Sam, the phone will alter it, but I can speak to Jake so that Sam will overhear.

"The children are screaming. The children need to be taken care of!" I blow smoke in Jake's face, while he whispers—he thinks Sam is on his side. He is fooled.

The children gather around my legs, and I say, "The children need attention! Who is taking care of the children?"

Sam has the message, and I cede control to him; I am to rest. I collapse at Jake's feet; I'm just a cloth doll, and now Sam is running things. When Jake hangs up, I arise, as if the breath of life has been blown back into the cloth.

Jake says I need to rest. I must comply and let the natural consequences of his control preside—the disorder that flows from evil. I lie on the bed, roll from side to side, but cannot sleep, hear a car honking, arise. In the kitchen, my ashtray fills. I do not empty it anymore but add to it, a mountain of butts, of ash, a memorial. Next to it sits a tiny vase with a mother and child protruding from its side, containing violets the children picked for me, now drooping. I place the flowers on the mountain of ash, now a shrine, flowers on the grave of my suffering, life juxtaposed with death, and arrange a few flowers in the form of a cross in front—the female symbol, the receptacle of ash, the fertile ground for flowers.

I cannot breathe in here. I must leave. I go outside, stand in the center of the street. There is no fear, no cars will come. I smoke, rock on my feet, centering.

Jake comes out and tries to force me back inside. I have smoked the last cigarette in the pack, only have my lighter for protection. He approaches me as I back into the street and flash my lighter.

"Don't you come near me. Stay away!"

But still he comes. So I flash it in his face, fighting fire with fire, and then throw the lighter at him, and run to the other side of the street. Is Sam still in the apartment above? I feel him protecting me.

Jake picks up the lighter and returns to the house. But I cannot leave him there alone. I must protect the children, must make him leave by staying. Maybe I must sleep with the Devil, offer myself up to him.

I enter the bedroom, now black as night. I lie down in darkness, on the Devil's pyre, the totem phalluses rising hugely from each corner of the bed. I am meant to sacrifice myself to the Devil—I lie with legs open, arms extended, like Jesus on the cross, but then clasp my hands above my head, forming a halo.

Is it Jake lying next to me? Or Sam? I carefully peek, but cannot tell for sure, so dark. As my eyes adapt, I see the wallpaper, the ribbons of orange and yellow, like flames arising out of hell. If I study the paper carefully, I can see men and women emerging from the flames, a pregnant woman facing one way becomes a man facing the other, but there are also tiny lines of gold woven through these bars of flame, the gold provided to protect me, countering the flames.

I notice an *S* scratched into the headboard above me—of course this is where we are to meet. It is not the Devil who is to make love to me here but Sam! I am a virgin on the pyre, and he will come to me in spirit, not in body, in this unholy hell—it will be our lovemaking that sanctifies, redeems, this hell.

I lie here and feel the gentle thrusts begin, his spirit moving into me; I, the Mother, he the Father. We join in the presence of evil—out of great evil arises great love. It is an immaculate conception, the merging of two spirits, and I am filled with wonder, with awe, that I have been chosen. Through me there will be a virgin birth, the birth of a new age, an age of love.

When it is over, I leave the room, sit, smiling, listening to the stereo. I see someone leave the bedroom and await Sam's appearance in the doorway. But it is Jake still. Maybe we may meet only in the world of spirit? Jake urges me to bed, but I say I am too happy to sleep. He disappears again, cannot bear my happiness.

CHAPTER 22:

RUNNING IN CIRCLES

Tuesday morning, 9/28. Jake says we must be at Sam's at seven thirty. I am not sure whether I am to leave the house—maybe we are really to meet here? The time has been filtered through the phone, so perhaps my role is to delay, to undermine Jake, a secret disruption.

When Donna arrives to watch the kids, I announce I must shower. Jake says, "There isn't time," and I say, "There is time," but then yield, don't shower, but change out of my sweatshirt. I must appear normal, as if the world is not altered. I choose a sweater, white for purity, with little flecks of blue and pink, still functional symbols but more discreet.

At Sam's, I am silent when he says hello. I am the nameless, the two of us are one, his hello reflects my inner hello—speech is unnecessary. When we are seated, I see Sam eyeing my auburn-colored purse. Something is wrong with it, he tells me with his eyes. I see it is open, the gold zipper, the protective gold gaping like an open mouth—this is supposed to be happening in secret, so I bend over, zip it up, and Sam leans back in relief. He peers at the pack of cigarettes I have tucked between my legs, and I immediately light up—he means I must continue to smoke. He starts to question us.

Jake says, "I think she needs help."

I smile. Sam knows I have all the help I need.

Sam asks me, "Have you been eating?"

"I've been drinking a lot of milk."

He nods—I have been right about doing that. "Have you been sleeping?"

"Jake would like me to sleep more, but I'm not tired." Meaning Jake would like me to sleep the big sleep, would like me to yield control, but I will not. I see that Sam's eyes are bloodshot, too, like mine. So tired.

"What's been happening?" he asks.

"I've been trying to let Jake run things around the house, and the house is just falling apart with disorder." The goal is to show that Jake is creating the chaos, to force him to take responsibility.

Jake says, "She's been acting erratic, not herself."

"In what way?"

But it is not to be said! I cross my legs tightly, and Jake is silent, I have shut him up. Then I recross my legs, and Jake crosses his leg in an opposing fashion. As he does this, Sam leans forward, and I see that his movement must compensate for the relative movement between Jake and me, so I carefully change my position. Jake adjusts his leg and Sam leans back. I don't know what to do to release Sam from this forced movement, so I glance at the door—should I leave?

Sam glances at the door, signaling me—there is too much power in here, too many mixed influences, and I must let Sam be in control.

I stand. "There's not enough air in here. I can't breathe. I need some fresh air."

Once outside the room, I think maybe he has wanted me to explore his house, that there's something I must discover. I walk down the hallway toward the bedroom, but Joy emerges. Sam must want me to constrain her influence, drive her out of the house, discreetly.

I turn and descend the stairs, walk in a circle on the landing, and Joy stands still, staring at me. Is she suspicious? Irritated that I am intervening? But it is Sam's wish, so I descend, circle the foyer, and leave the house. If I stay, Joy will leave, so I sit on the steps. Joy walks around me and down the steps, toward her car, while I, with my cigarette, direct her to leave.

When she is gone, I move into the street and stare up at the therapy room, focusing my power on it, then form a cross by walking in front of the house, sanctifying his space. I am about to circle the house when Jake emerges. Sam waves as we leave—all is well, proceeding according to plan.

A little later, Sam calls. I lift the receiver.

"Linda?"

"Hmmm," I say, like "Om," a meditation—I am to be silent.

"I've arranged a meeting for you and Jake with Dr. Morton at seven thirty this evening."

It is a folding in of time, reflecting our morning meeting of seven thirty, and it must be that Sam and I are to meet through intermediaries—we cannot meet directly.

He continues, "I moved heaven and earth to arrange this meeting, so please do your best to be on time."

I smile at his humor, that he has moved heaven and earth. But maybe both Sam and I are merely disciples, and Dr. Morton, this "good man, good person," is a higher-up, our superior. Or merely another disciple? Maybe there are six or eight people in the world working simultaneously to effect the change.

Sam gives me directions, but he is speaking too fast. I merely write words that I pick out here and there, but it does not matter—I am not meant to leave the house at all; he is telling me the reverse of what he means. I am not to go, not to be on time. I am to stay exactly where I am.

"Do you understand the directions?" he asks.

"Yes, I do understand. Let me tell Jake." I place the receiver to my heart. He must hear my heart beating.

Jake's mother, Teri, arrives.

Jessie protests, "Don't go! I don't want to stay with Nana."

Teri grabs her by the shoulders, and Jessie spins around and strikes out at her, and says, "I hate you!"

Teri snaps, "These children are out of control. They need to be taught to respect their elders. Jessie's mouth should be washed out with soap. If they were my children—"

"Well, they are not your children." I move close to her face and say, "Why is it that you don't like my children? You don't love them—why do you expect them to stay with you?"

Taken aback, Teri grabs their jackets and says to Jake, "I'll take them to the park."

Jake is helping with the jackets, and I pretend to help, but Teri is trying to take the children away from me. No way am I going to let that happen, so when Teri is first to walk out the door, I quickly shut it, automatically locking it. But there are two locks, protective gold. They have protected me all along. A gold key projects from the top lock, the deadbolt. I turn it for good measure and take out the key.

Jake, who has gone to get his jacket, comes up behind me and yells, "What are you doing?"

"The children are staying with me," I say, as he jiggles the door handle. He sees the key in my hand and grabs it, unlocks the deadbolt, steps out, holds the screen door open and calls to the kids.

I block the kids' exit and close the door, locking Jake out too. Just as Joy has been driven out of Sam's house, so my role is to drive Jake out.

Jake and Teri each try the door handle, and I stand silently behind the door until I see them leave, heading for the back door, which is open, I remember almost too late. I race to it and lock it twice, removing the gold, the key.

Then Jake and Teri are at the front door again, yelling, "Let us in!"

"Mumma—let them in! Please, Mumma," Jessie says, while Brandon sucks his thumb, looking tearful.

I must do as the children wish, so I unlock the front door but make a point of putting the wrong key into the lock, reserving the other one, the gold, in my pocket. Jake is already locked out anyway, metaphorically—I am protected with my watch of gold, the blue elastic band threaded with gold that holds my hair, and even my cigarette pack with its gold band. But there is also silver foil, so I remove it, separating the gold from the silver. I am gold, Jake is silver, his silver ring, his silver bracelet—all along there have been these signs.

It is not Jake driving the car, Jake is only our puppet, he has no control. I am Sam's eyes, he receives my words through the radio and drives via Jake, and I must relay to him all that I see. So much responsibility. "We are approaching a stop sign . . . There is a car turning in front of us . . . Slow down, step on the brakes . . . We are now on Mount Auburn Street, passing the cemetery . . . The light is green, you can go . . ." and so on. But how can I continue speaking nonstop? What if my voice gives out?

Finally, finally, we arrive at what is supposed to be Dr. Morton's house. Or is it really Sam's and my house? Is Dr. Morton there to restrain Jake? To make Sam's and my meeting possible?

We walk a flagstone path through a garden. A fountain, a boy peeing, is just visible in the darkness. Returning to the Garden, the beginning of all time.

We pass through two doors to enter the foyer, the foyer enclosed twice, the door fixtures gold, a sign. The foyer is under construction, an apparently new door to the left, a door to the right. The construction—reality in a transitional state. As we enter, we face a mantel, an altar separating the two doors.

Dr. Morton invites us in. I circle around the overhead light in the foyer, then enter the room to the right with Jake. We sit, facing Dr. Morton. I note his bloodshot eyes, his *well-traveled* eyes, and am assured he is a fellow worker/prophet who has not been allowed sleep either.

He observes me. I must be very careful, the balance of the world depends on it. I must not reveal what I know, the changes we are attempting to make. Must pretend that all is well, manage the presence of evil with nonchalance, delicately, carefully. If the meeting progresses well, it will be Jake who is identified as the perpetrator of chaos, the one who needs help. I am delivering him into their hands so he may be constrained from continuing his evil. Dr. Morton will separate him from me, making the critical meeting possible, my union with Sam.

He questions me about the usual—sleeping, eating—and pretends I am the patient, but really is seeking reassurance I am able to persist with our shared struggle.

"I'm doing what I can under the circumstances—"

Jake interrupts, "She seems to be lost in her own world. I'm concerned."

I smile—better my world than his.

Dr. Morton watches me for a moment but cannot maintain eye contact—I must be shining so brightly it hurts his eyes. Is it not odd that Jake does not notice the light emanating from me? He, too, cannot look at me for long, but the difference is that he is unconscious of why he cannot maintain his gaze, while Morton knows. I wonder about our roles, whether Morton and I are peers, he my superior, or I his.

"I'd like to speak with Jake alone, if I may," he says.

I nod. He is preparing the situation for my meeting with Sam. He glances out the window. I can just barely see the fountain—he must want me to go outside.

"Just for a few minutes," he says, meaning there is little time in which to find Sam, but he will do his best.

I leave the room. In the foyer, I am to explore, to find Sam's true home. Maybe if I step through the newly constructed door, not the entrance, I will enter an alternative reality. I open the door to a space that may exist in another time/space dimension and peer in, find a desk. It might be Sam's, but he is not there.

I step outside. Maybe if I stand in the dark, peer into the light, it will be Sam in the window with his friend, not Jake. I walk near the fountain, turn, and see Jake and Dr. Morton inside, but they don't see me, the moon, in the dark, revolving outside the window.

They call me inside. Dr. Morton says he is going to prescribe some medication that will help me sleep. He looks at me pointedly and asks, "Any questions?"

He is providing the medication to appease Jake, pretending it is I who need help. But I gather from his eyes, the care with which he gazes at me, that I am not really supposed to take the pills. I am to do the reverse of what is spoken, the truth revealed in silence only, in the nonverbal sphere. And I certainly must not sleep—we are approaching the critical moment! I say I understand. We shake hands and I feel him transmitting a supportive energy.

Once home, after a stop at the drugstore, I pretend to take a pill, but as I do, I spin around and spit it into the glass of water, and quickly pour it out into the sink.

"You didn't take it!" Jake accuses.

"You're the one who needs it. I don't need it."

I drop the bottle in the trash, but he immediately retrieves it and sets it on the counter. How to dispose of it? Jessie calls out from the bedroom, and when Jake leaves the kitchen, I take the pills into the pantry and drop them through the slit window screen to the concrete driveway below, the little white pills splattering among the drops of white paint/semen. Jake comes up behind me as I stand near the window.

"What have you done with the pills?"

"I threw them out," I say, inadvertently letting a little smile escape as I turn to the window, so that he follows my gaze to the concrete below.

He runs outside, retrieves the pills, and again tries to make me take them.

"You want me to eat these shards of plastic? No way will I take that into my body!"

He sets the broken container on the counter.

Triavil, I read—isn't that an antidepressant? Bizarre. I have never before felt so good, have never been less depressed in my life, so elated.

Jake whispers on the phone, as if I won't understand, then hangs up, saying he has arranged a meeting with Sam tomorrow morning, Wednesday morning.

"I don't need to see Sam," I say, but I am secretly pleased.

This has been the plan all along, I intuit, that it will be Jake, the Devil incarnate, who arranges our meeting, the critical day, Weds-day. It's about time—I don't know how long I can go on smoking nonstop, keeping this little light burning, following the multitude of cues, so hard having to be everywhere at once, responsible for everything, generating the energy to keep the world from falling into catastrophe.

CHAPTER 23:

RAGGEDY DOLL, ARISE

Wednesday morning, 9/29. As we near Donna's house, I see a car parked in front of a neighbor's house, with a man and woman inside, making out, the woman gaudy with makeup—they are like animals having sex, exposed in that car. They look up and glare at me, and I turn, exude energy through my eyes, trying to overcome this evil, this animal passion exposed for all to view.

Jake takes the kids inside, and when he returns and opens his car door, I get out, a symbolic refusal to reside within the same space, and when he gets out too, I climb back in. Finally we are both in the car.

"Take me home now!" I insist, but he refuses. But I must return home! Stay to leave, stay to leave. It is at home that Sam and I are to meet.

As Jake inserts the key in the ignition, I remember Sam removing the key from his car, and I grab the key, pull, and it breaks in the ignition. I rejoice, but Jake is angry.

"What are you doing?!"

He fiddles around and removes the broken key. He holds out his hand and says, "Give me yours, c'mon!"

I hand it to him. Maybe this is the point—my key in the ignition, my key running the car.

We drive, and I open my purse, the gold zipper like Sam's teeth, the purse open to release his influence, his symbolic voice, and I frantically rummage through the purse, find items with protective gold: keys, hairbands woven with gold, my cigarette pack. They have a certain power—I can alter our course with them. It is critical whether they are in or out of the bag, whether the zipper is open or shut. This is why Sam has repeatedly eyed my purse, indicating its power. I discreetly rearrange the items. If I do it right, we will not go to Sam's office at the hospital. We will, to Jake's surprise, end up at home, where I am to meet Sam.

But to my own surprise, we arrive at the hospital. It must be the plan. We enter the hospital through a door that has not been there before; the whole wing has been altered—Sam has created the illusion of Belmont Hospital for Jake's benefit and altered his memory so he does not realize it has been changed. As we enter, I read a sign, a red sign, NO SMOKING, a white cross in a circle barring a smoking cigarette. Red, meaning do the opposite, so I light up, circle in front of the sign, sanctifying the space, while Jake approaches an information desk, also not there before.

We find Sam's room. It appears the same, a sanctuary of sameness within all that has been altered. He wears his auburn suit, the color that symbolizes our union, and I smile, as we sit in our swivel chairs. I carefully set my purse on the floor, and Sam eyes it—it must have been a dangerous move, so I pick it up again, hold it in my lap, test whether it should be open or closed by observing his reactions. I swivel and then Jake swivels in reaction, and Sam leans forward, and I see I must continue counteracting Jake's movements, attempting to allow Sam relief from his consequent contortions.

Sam's eyes are also bloodshot, so tired still, and still I am pivotal. I try to adjust my movements—there is this constant reordering of their bodies depending on what I do. There is too much power in this room, and I think that if I feign collapse, Sam can assume power, so I make myself limp, while Sam speaks. When he speaks to me, I abruptly come alive, a cloth doll surging with life. I realize we must proceed as if all is normal, as if the world has not changed.

Sam asks me how I'm doing.

"*I'm* fine," I say, implying that Jake has gone wild. "But just look at me, wearing these smelly shirts. Jake wouldn't let me shower, change, or even put on my makeup. And he wouldn't let me eat or sleep—I must have lost seven or eight pounds already." Thinking, the tables are to be turned, reality rotated so Jake emerges as the one who needs to change.

Sam nods—I am proceeding correctly. He says he and Jake will walk me downstairs to see if I can be admitted. "If you won't take the medication, I have to admit you."

I nod. I see. I have done correctly by not taking the medication, and now we will pretend to take me to the psychiatric department, at which time Jake will be institutionalized. We will lure him there in this way.

We start to walk, and Sam takes my hand! He holds it firmly. Jake walks on my left, Sam on my right, but it is Sam who holds my hand. We are allies. We touch—I am so glad finally to be held. But as we walk, I must stop at all the red signs, stop, circle, go, smoke, and let go of Sam's hand. He waits as I consecrate our little procession, sanctify the halls, then takes my hand again, until we enter a small room.

There is an examining table, a chair across from it, a step stool, a sink, and a multitude of medical equipment. Sam leaves, returns with other men, a doctor and a social worker, and they speak to me. When Sam speaks, I become limp, a cloth doll; we are one, and only one of us can have control at a time. I become his cloth doll, his living phobia that will not hurt him after all, but that assists him, liberates him from his fear. The doll becomes limp, the doll comes alive, the doll dies so he can live, the doll lives so he may rest. They think I am merely tired, but I am feigning this to give Sam his rightful power.

When it is my turn to speak, I abruptly sit up straight, answer whatever question, then relax my muscles, slump into a pile of cloth, my head sinking to my chest. The doctor asks me to get onto the examining table, and a stool is placed between my chair and the table, and they tell me to be very careful. I gather I am not to touch the floor—something terrible might happen. Maybe to Sam, who is no longer in the room? I carefully place my feet on the stool, make it to the table, the floor untouched—I must not let him die. They take my blood pressure; I am a stand-in for Sam. Does his heart still beat? I represent the two of us. Are we alive?

A nurse brings in some orange juice she wants me to drink. But I know what is in the orange juice, so I lift the cup to my lips, wander over to the sink, and discreetly dump it and hand the cup back. The nurse brings me another orange juice, and the next time, I dump it through a crack in the examining table, where it forms a pool on the floor they cannot see.

Food is brought in on a cart. Chicken salad sandwiches, custard.

"Jake, why don't you eat, you haven't eaten in a long time." I serve him, smiling, and he eats. He can eat of this vile world. My back turned, I dump my own food in the trash.

Jake does not let me get too close to the door, but while he eats, I weasel my way around him and check behind the curtain to see if I can move the glass door. When it moves, I walk out, but Jake quickly grabs my arm and pulls me back into the room. I am furious. We have been here far too long.

"Take me home! If you don't take me home this minute, I'll divorce you!" I swing my shoulder bag at him, hitting him in the stomach, and then he reaches for me, but I grab his arms.

He quickly pulls away. "You scratched me!"

"I hate you. I hate you. Take me home. Take me home, or I'll divorce you!"

Then he is gone, and standing at the door are two male security guards, in uniform, who pretend I am not there.

Where is Sam? I look through the glass and there he is. I can just make him out in a bed across the hall, dying. Of a heart attack? There is an oxygen mask on his face—what must I do to save him? Frantically, I look around the room, see tubes hanging from the wall, marked OXYGEN. I am to blow through the tubes, send my breath to him, the breath of life. He is the one in need now. The reverse of my dream of the Asian doctor blowing in my face to help me quit smoking. I fiddle with the tubes, but when I look, Sam's bed is no longer there.

I say I have to pee. The guard walks me to a restroom, but he will not shut the restroom door. He expects me to pee with the door ajar, but I cannot, so I just sit clothed on the toilet. I see a black rubber circle on the wall, metal in the center, an observing eye masked as a doorstop, so I crouch low. They must not see me here. I flush the toilet, feeling the discomfort of my swollen bladder. Piles of supplies line the wall, and I quickly try to rearrange the rolls of toilet paper so they too sit below the gaze of the electric eye, but the door opens, and I must go back.

I am in the room again, and it is changed. Jake pokes his head in, and I ask him what has happened to the room, and he says they have removed some of the medical equipment, that they were concerned I might damage it. *Might damage their plan*, I think. I see there are outlets in here, too, little discreet holes in the wall—I must not walk in front of them, it will disrupt the electromagnetic waves. I must not let myself be seen. Then too there are signs, DANGER, OXYGEN, and DO NOT SMOKE, but I am dying for a cigarette, and I say, "Please, can I smoke somewhere?" and the guard says sure. I ask about the signs, and the guard says the oxygen has been turned off. I crouch below the invisible rays that crisscross the room, a second ceiling cutting the room in half, and huddle in a corner and smoke.

I am not sure whether the guards are here to protect me from Jake, are surrogates for Sam, or are there to constrain me. I walk to the door, bent below the rays, and look out. There is an emergency exit to the left, and that must be the way I am to leave—it says DO NOT ENTER: FOR EMERGENCY USE ONLY, and I deduce that the reverse is true. It is a camouflage for Jake's sake, my way out—maybe Sam is waiting for me to make my move.

I am pondering what to do when Sam returns with a nurse and tells me to drink the juice, that there is medication in it that will be helpful. I do it, trusting him—it is part of the plan. I say I need to go to the bathroom, but they will not let me go by myself. They expect me to pee while a man is watching me. The nurse says she will accompany me, and finally I get to go, the second time, twice.

I see Sam across the hallway, making phone calls, trying to find a place for me, working within this context, which is evil, run by Jake's crew, the nurses everywhere, the police. He stands there within view, one piece of goodness that will not leave me here, that I can count on. Is he actually trying to work out where to place Jake? When will I ever be able to leave this room? I have been here forever. When I ask the guards the time, I discover it has been almost eight hours.

Finally Sam comes, with Jake, and says he has found a place for me at Mount Auburn, that Belmont has no room, and Jake will drive me there. Jake asks for an ambulance instead, but Sam says, "All will be well," and I see I am to allow Jake to deliver me. Perhaps Jake will unknowingly take me to Sam's and my home.

Sam takes my hand, walks with us all the way to the car. My ally.

CHAPTER 24:

RETURN TO THE WOMB, WITH EMERGENCY EXIT

Once again I am surprised when Jake and I end up at our pretended destination, Mount Auburn Hospital. I realize the name—auburn—is a sign. It is Sam's hospital. It is here we will meet.

After an interview in which I speak clearly, reasonably about Jake's behavior in relation to me—I must make them see it is he who must be hospitalized—I am walked to another floor and Jake says goodbye. Finally I am free of him.

In the staff office, my blood pressure is taken—they want to make sure I can continue—and a man named Fred asks for my purse. I search his eyes, and finding them bloodshot (well-traveled) like Sam's and mine, I know he is an ally, and so I hand it over. Carefully, he removes its contents, sorts through the powerful objects, removing the gold (the keys) and the silver (nail clippers, Swiss Army knife). He will keep them in a safe place for me—they have been awaiting the delivery of these magic wands.

A woman dressed in street clothes, maybe not a nurse, walks me to my room and asks if I'd like some food. It feels safe to eat here, so I order an egg salad sandwich.

I study the room. It is not a hospital room after all but a home, Sam's and my room. Two beds, his shoes (leather oxfords), his books on a bedside table, an apple (an unadulterated apple sitting there, a comic clue), and a blue suitcase. Perhaps he has just arrived? And there are balls of yarn and flowers. So comfortable. Maybe he really works here and this room is reserved for him, his secret home. Maybe no one is to know we will live here together.

When the food arrives, I eat, then hide the containers under some hospital gowns. No one must know I am here. I cannot leave the room.

I examine the book on the table nearest me, open it to the middle, and start to read. I am astonished to read of my great aunt Erma. It is the story of my family right here in this book, as if it had all been written long ago, and only now am I privy to its contents. Is this heaven where all of the past and future is known? Why has the book been left for me to read? I see the words through a haze, the words to the left and right lost in blurred light, and as I read, the words become visible. I become increasingly amused—it is as if the words are being written as I read, tongue in cheek, teasing me. They are clues to what I must do so Sam may enter. I read: *She peered out the window.*

So I look out the window, see mop or broom handles through the window of a neighboring room. Am I to prepare the room? I see now that male and female items are intermixed, so I separate them, the shoes on his side, the yarn on mine. Open the suitcase, find it empty, place my purse inside, the auburn of it, Sam enclosed in it symbolically. Tuck the teddy bear on the other bed under the covers—Sam may now sleep with me.

The door opens and someone peeks inside, then shuts the door. They want to make sure I am okay and have not been discovered. Is there some other exit I am to take? Two doors to the armoire, with gold keys protruding. If I pass through one of the doors, will I pass into another reality? The right door is open, only clothing and hangers inside. I crawl into the left side, a small space, but nothing happens, so I step out again. I examine the entrance to the room, see both silver and gold hardware, mixed cues—I'm unsure whether I am to pass through.

The knob turns—someone is at the door. I must not be seen. I hold my breath, stand behind the door. A woman enters, gazes around the room, looks at me and raises her eyebrows, but says nothing. She undresses, crawls into bed, places her hands on her chest, and shuts her eyes, does not move. I cannot even see her breathe. She is a living corpse, her face a skull, her arms so thin they are merely bone.

Why is she lying in Sam's bed? Am I meant to imitate her? Is she demonstrating what to do? The plan: I must pretend to be dead, and then I will be taken from here on a bier, taken to Sam. I crawl under the covers, arrange them so my clothes do not show, only my head protrudes. I, too, place my hands over my heart, pretend I lie in a casket or on my deathbed, do not move, take shallow breaths. Someone is at the door. My eyes are shut. I do not breathe. The door closes. I wait, but no one comes—they think I merely sleep. Maybe this is not his room after all?

I arise, go to the door. Perhaps I am to walk out. I tentatively step out, pressing my body against the wall, outside the cones of light that dot the hall. I eye the room directly across from mine—perhaps it is in this reflection of my room that he sleeps. I edge toward it and slowly open the door. I sigh with relief—Brandon lies there with his teddy in one bed; he is safe, with me after all. In the other bed, I cannot see too clearly, but surely it is Sam, and he is wearing tight short pajama bottoms—they are a child's clothes, a message for me to grow up; he must remain a child as long as I do.

I am angry at his twisted humor, and yell, "Fuck you!" into the darkness and slam the door. *Fuck you* because he thinks we must remain separated, the boys and the girls, until I grow up, when it is he who is wearing children's clothes.

I return to my room, and it is Jessie's dark hair lying across the pillow of the other bed. Thank God, the children are safe here with me. Thank God. Now I can sleep.

I am told breakfast is being served, I must come out to the dining room, but I say I am not hungry, I am tired. But the woman does not want me to sleep, still I am not allowed to sleep, so I comply.

There are women and a few men sitting around the long table. I circle the lights and enclose the table, walk around it clockwise, then counterclockwise, twice to enclose. They say I must eat, so I conclude I am not to eat.

A woman loudly proclaims, "Louise can't see. She can't see . . ." I go to the window—is there something I am meant to see? Am I the eyes? Or are these people blinded by my light and truly cannot see me? I am safe here, unseen—when I look, no one looks directly at me. I must appear to be a blaze of light, my cigarette glowing, a radiance that hides me.

A man and a woman take me to a small room. They cannot meet my eyes. I must look different to them than I appear to myself. A man and a woman—the hospital cannot distinguish my sex, so they provide one of each. They glance surreptitiously at my body and then away, as if I am naked, though I see I am clothed. I pick up my purse to cover my apparent nudity, my genitals, and cross my arms. I am androgynous, nude, an oddity, but they try to act casual, as if nothing is unusual.

They ask the dates of my children's births. I take my time, then carefully say: April 3, 1978, and May 20, 1980. I'm sure I'm right, but still they cannot look at me, and then I realize—I am a ghost, a phantom from the past intruding into the future. They ask me these dates to determine the time from which I come. Although I am sure I am correct, they are astonished, these dates from a century or so ago, but they hide their amazement, and now I understand why they cannot look at me—I am just a haze, a distant whispering voice, or I am decaying flesh rotting on blackened bones, and there is a smell they cannot tolerate, although they try to hide their discomfort.

Even though I can see I am clothed, not nude, this must be a conjunction of realities, a crack in some time warp that I have slipped through, and what appears to be true is differently perceived from each side of the time warp. I speak slowly; it is so hard to form the words, as if the words take time to pass through the ages separating us. I am male and female, a goddess of sorts, a source of light, and they are careful, reverent. They must not look into my eyes, the light shining so brightly.

They escort me through the hall, eye my purse, signaling me that I need to cover myself in this reality, and I move the purse to cover my genitals once again. I walk into a room. There is a TV in it, a white-haired woman lounging, her feet up on a table, another woman on the other side.

I look in my purse, but my cigarettes are not there. I see them lying near the woman with white hair. I look directly at her and she acknowledges me with her eyes—yes, those are the cigarettes I am to smoke. I cautiously approach her, watching her eyes. Am I doing right? But the woman turns to talk to her neighbor. I take a cigarette, lift the lighter—the lighter has words on it: "The Best Man for the Job Is a Woman"—and it must be my lighter, it's obviously meant for me, man-woman. I pick up the pack, the lighter, and deposit them in my purse. The woman is still looking the other way, pretending not to notice. But she has supplied me, so must be my ally.

I need to use the bathroom, so I weave out of the room. I face two bathrooms, one says WOMEN and the other, MEN, but with a handmade sign above it saying WOMEN. It is the bathroom provided for me, the androgyne. I enter, and to the right is a cubicle, but there is another door in front of me, a room within a room, two bathrooms, the second one an addition. I enter the second. I am being observed through an electric eye on the wall, so gross. I flush the toilet, then see the other cubicle.

I must go twice, two aspects, the man and the woman, and I mimic peeing the second time.

In the cubicle are both silver fixtures and gold hangers. To counteract the silver with the gold, I arrange a hanger atop the silver toilet paper holder. As I flush a second time and leave, I notice a sign on the door: PLEASE CHECK TWICE TO MAKE SURE YOU HAVE NOT LEFT ANY PERSONAL ARTICLES. Twice, the significant clue, and I flush the first toilet, shut that door again, then flush the second toilet, rearrange the hangers, and shut that cubicle door again. With a sigh of relief, I leave the bathroom, then reopen the door, shut it. Twice. Twice to enclose, twice to enfold.

I am taken to another room where I find objects under construction, in different phases of completion. I am asked to sit with the others at the table, meaning I am to sit apart. I climb onto a tall swivel chair, where I can rotate, orchestrate what goes on. The old woman says, "Louise can't see, she can't see . . ." I must see for her; I am the eyes, invisible to them—they cannot see me as I direct the action. I light up a cigarette.

The white-haired woman points at me. "She has my cigarettes!" And then to me, "Give them back!"

I must pretend to comply. I rise, approach her, my hand out, but then turn, put the cigarettes back into my purse, and climb back onto my stool, where I resume rotating, smoking. I notice a smell of incense in the room, signaling Sam's presence, the Eastern influence.

Another woman enters the room, sniffs the air. "What's that smell?" She looks out onto a porch accessible through a door at the back of the room, before eyeing me and saying, "You can't smoke in here. Put your cigarette out."

I get off the stool, but must keep my cigarette burning, and I carry it "out" onto the porch.

"Come back here!"

I take this to mean I am moving in the right direction, always doing the opposite—that is the key.

But the woman grasps my arm and escorts me back into the room where the others wait. They are discussing jobs for the week, who is in charge of which things: the Kleenex, the ashtrays, kitchen cleanup, and finally, turning off the television. This last duty clarifies the time frame, the difference in our realities. I have noticed the TV is not turned off in the usual manner. There is some futuristic skill involved, something telepathic—there are no buttons in evidence. The assignments acknowledge the significance of concrete objects.

I am urged to eat again. They are testing me, and I refuse, but I am out of cigarettes, and they say I can have one if I eat. I must continue smoking until Sam comes for me, my only protection, and so I eye the food. All I allow myself is the custard—white, pure. I drink my milk.

A big woman, with long auburn-colored hair, talks to me in a loud voice. I search her eyes, find them bloodshot, the way I can identify our compatriots, the friends of our great cause, so I follow her. As she speaks in her big voice, she glances behind herself periodically, so I gather her speech is intended as a diversion to deceive other staff members.

She guides me to the men's/women's bathroom, sneaks me in there. I watch her eyes to see if I am doing what is desired. As I pass the first cubicle, I see a flash of rust-colored clothing under it, so I know Sam is there. But there is some ritual we must proceed through before we can meet. I look toward the second cubicle and look back at the woman, who nods, yes, talking all the while, telling me to get undressed—she wants me to shower.

I do these things wordlessly—I must not speak. A ritual preparation. After my shower, she holds robes for me and puts them on me backward, as if I am backward. She leads me toward the door.

I glance at the other cubicle, look at her, but now she wants me to leave. Maybe Sam has to go through the same ritual before we meet. I weave around the lights, but still he does not come. I cannot find him anywhere.

In the main hall I see a door I have not noticed before: EMERGENCY EXIT: DO NOT OPEN, and I think it is my door, only I am to open it. But it is not an emergency, and I am to do the opposite of the signs. I reach out and push the door, will simply walk out to meet him. As I push, there is an ear-shattering buzz, a siren, and I stand back in astonishment. People are running toward me, and someone is yelling, "Turn off the buzzer!"

I am taken to a tiny room containing a cot. I lie down. Fred, the big guy who removed the special items from my purse, sits reading a newspaper in a chair that blocks the doorway. The paper says Friday, October 1, but I cannot see the year. They do not want me to leave this room. People pass by, look in, but seem not to see me. Maybe there is a shield of sorts that renders me invisible, or maybe I appear only as a dim light. They keep me in this small place—maybe it is a secret place so no one will know I am here; maybe it appears different from outside the room than from within it.

If only I could discover the year. Maybe time is now flowing backward; maybe I am growing smaller, receding into childhood, infancy. I am not to speak; I am speechless, an infant. There is something I want badly, my body aches for it, a cigarette maybe, but babies don't smoke, I am not even to smoke, and I lie here whining, a baby murmuring in need, and I am growing smaller, and smaller, and maybe I am returning to the womb, this small tight place, and then receding further, returning to the nothingness before I ever was. *Oh please, Sam, don't let me die here, please, Sam, come to me, where are you, I am your child, please come to me*, and I whine, and the man looks, moves his leg, tips his chair, and I no longer know what it all means.

Another night passes. It is morning, and Sam finally comes.

He shakes my hand, shakes it again, twice I feel him squeeze, and it is as if he pulls me through time, through the haze, and then we are walking to another room. Inside, the chairs are strangely skewed, as if the room has tipped, pushing the chairs into tight concentric circles around the window, through which the sun shines. We are in the audience of God, Sam and me in an empty room, the halls full of people who cannot follow us, as in my dream. As we sit here, I cannot tell which shines brighter, Sam or the sun, or are they the same, shining on each side of me? I cannot look at him for long—he is too bright.

He is talking to me about another facility, a place with locked doors, because I have tried to leave. They do not feel they can contain me here. Do I understand?

Of course, I think, they cannot contain me—how can they contain pure light? Invisibility? I have achieved what I started out to do, to leave by staying. I say, "I only opened the door, I didn't walk through it." I laugh a little.

"It was a fire door," he says. There is a grimace on his face, as if I have done something wrong. He says he knows some of the staff at Charles River and that it's a good private hospital.

I think perhaps his words are merely a cover-up, maybe there are people who might overhear, who listen from another room, and in reality he will be taking me home, to our home. He grasps my hand again, squeezing it twice, a secret handshake.

CHAPTER 25:

HE LOVES ME, HE LOVES ME NOT

The man drives, and the woman suggests that I lie down on a bed in the back of the ambulance, a secret way of getting me out. I ask whether they would like me to strap myself in, but they say it is not necessary. They have the radio on, pretend they are not acting, are very casual, as if this were not the critical event that it is, but are meanwhile listening for cues on the radio—it is WMJX, Sam's frequency.

I look out the window. They are driving in an unexpected direction, a distorted route to Sam's home, a camouflage of our journey to lead anyone astray who might be following.

But no. We arrive, not at Sam's, but in some beautiful country setting, an arboretum of sorts, and stop in front of a red brick building.

Sunday, 10/3, early. Sam comes. I am still in my nightgown, which Jake dropped off with some other things the day before. With no other private place available, we have to meet in my room. I sit on my bed, while he pulls up a chair. He is wearing a golf shirt, a little alligator on his pocket, pretending to be my parent, my father who golfs, my mother who golfs—how can he be a golfer? Is it a necessary pretense? Or a cruel joke, a betrayal?

"Why are you wearing that shirt?"

"I enjoy a round of golf every now and then. In fact, I'm on my way there now."

"It's Sunday—why are you here?" I look at him, but then turn my head away. "I can't look at you, you're too bright."

"Then look away," he says rather abruptly, and I look out the window to my left.

He sits quietly, and I am silent. Finally, he says, "What are you thinking right now?"

I decide to simply say it. "We should be lovers."

"Linda, I'm your therapist."

"Yes." I shrug. So what?

When he leaves, leaving me there, I can hardly believe it. How can this be?

Jake brings the kids, and I am so happy to see them. I love them so much. They have brought me pictures they have colored, which I tape above my bed.

We descend to the dining room. The children are wild, all over the place, wanting to snack on cookies, drink milk. In minutes, a pile of empty cellophane, paper sleeves torn from straws, and napkins gradually appear on the table, sprinkled with spilled milk and sugar packets. It is so exhausting that already I cannot wait for them to leave.

Jake says he has talked to my father, who is unsure about whether to call me, so perhaps I should call him? I am thinking about whether I will be able to find change to make a call, whether I can figure out how to use the pay phone, whether I will have the energy to lift the receiver, to speak, when Jake says that Sam has called my mother and reassured her that what I'm going through is not the same as Brian, that it is something different. While I see why he might say such a thing, I also am a little angry—how can he possibly know?

Donna, Sara, and Bea come too, and I shuffle to greet them, say hello, but cannot make my face smile though I am happy they have come. So hard to speak, to form words, to respond in time. I am so slow, the whole world is slowed for me, yet I cannot keep up with it. It is the drugs. I am locked up twice, inside the locked doors, inside the drugs.

I break my virtual silence, ask the staff questions: How can I get out? I am told I can sign a three-day paper, *AMA*, Against Medical Advice, if necessary, and then I can leave. Staff explain the complications, but it is so confusing. I say I just want to go home, and I sign the paper.

The next time Sam comes, he is angry. Why have I signed a three-day? If I don't retract it, he will have to have me committed, a complicated legal process, and it will be even harder for me to leave. I realize then that I must demonstrate I deserve to be free, that I am going to have to work for it. Climb the little ladder of privileges to gain my freedom. Comply with everything. I retract the three-day.

I take my medication, the nurse always observing closely—she does not trust me. I learn their names: Haldol, Cogentin, more each time. It is difficult to walk. I shuffle—what I will later call the Haldol shuffle, holding my hands up in front of me like a squirrel, as if they are paws, fingers limp, wrists stiff. It is hard to smile, to move my facial muscles, as if I have been coated in cement, hard to speak, too, and there is no chair, no bed that is comfortable. Is the discomfort intentional?

We are not allowed to lie in our rooms—there are endless activities so we may not think too much, to keep us talking, moving, involved. I cannot keep the activities straight, try to record the schedule in my notebook so I know where to be, but I can barely write. It is the writing of an old person, jerky, jagged lines, broken—why can't I write my usual rounded letters?

Sam comes. There is no office available, so we go to another empty room, with a single bed in it and what appears to be a two-way mirror. Are we being observed? I sit on the bed, and then move over so Sam can sit, but he pulls over a chair I hadn't noticed. I am a little embarrassed about my maneuver but say nothing.

He asks me the meaning of certain proverbs: "People who live in glass houses shouldn't throw stones," "A rolling stone gathers no moss," "Still waters run deep." I try to answer, knowing this is a test, but fumble my words. He shakes his head in discouragement.

We talk a while, slowly, quietly, and then he leans toward me, his hands folded together, his eyes zeroing in on my eyes, and I hear him saying something, almost whispering—it sounds as if he has rehearsed it; it doesn't sound like him, not the Sam I know. His brows are knitted, his eyes squinting, as if he is in pain. I can't hear him clearly.

He repeats the words, "And when you realized I didn't love you, was not in love with you?"

I take a breath, but burst into tears, sobbing—I cannot, cannot, believe what he is saying. "Why are you saying this? How can you say this? You're the only person who cares . . ."

I weep all the way through our handshake. Why didn't he tell me that before?! Why couldn't he have said it long ago? Now I am going to have to fight my way out of here. It is all up to me. It is my struggle. I am actually locked up in a mental institution. I am going to have to fight for my mind, to recover it.

Hours later, alone, I tear up when I think of what Sam said about not loving me but then recall his odd introductory phrase, "And when you realized . . ." Why had he pretended I already understood his feelings, when I did not? When he knew I didn't? He had whispered it, maybe knowing he had to say something to break my obsession, but at the same time, perhaps trying not to lie, he made it a statement from my supposed point of view.

And what about that iffy mirror—had we been observed? Did someone tell him he needed to say this?

But enough. I see I must free myself from this futile entanglement—Sam's feelings, real or unreal, are irrelevant after all. I can't really know. What I must remember: He has said what he won't do.

I struggle through the paralysis of the drugs, befriend the other patients, the friendless. I sit in the dining room smoking, my long hair lank, curving onto the table surface, my face clear, no cosmetics, my eyelashes invisible, my skin pale.

A young man shuffles up to me. His hands hide in his pockets, pulling his pants dangerously low, his underwear peeking out. People continually remind him: *Pull up your pants, Bobby.* He is an abased version of me, a reflection, with his long wispy, greasy hair, bloated features, mottled skin. One of the more frightening patients. He hangs around me, drawn to me over and over again.

Finally he says, "Have you been to heaven? You look as though you've been to heaven."

I can see myself through his eyes: androgynous face, the sadness, the long hair, the delicately thin body—Jesus, I look like Jesus. With a smile, a little laugh, I say, "Yes, to a heaven of sorts, not what you think."

He pulls a picture of himself, pre-Thorazine, out of his wallet, and I see that once he was remarkably good-looking, a young man with his life still before him, sitting on a pillow, holding his guitar. Then he opens his mouth and sings to me, and a hush falls over the cafeteria. The shock of Bobby singing. The shock of Bobby coming out of his haze.

Endless meetings. Social skills group ("If you were an animal, what animal would you be?" "What color?" Intellectually patronizing, but fun, easy to identify who has written which answers—I am a bird, purple), community meeting, module meeting, women's group, planning meeting, group therapy, couples group, individual therapy, etc., all in different rooms, with different people.

I am so helpful to other group members with my insights that I rise to the position of patient-therapist, not quite identified with either. I monitor my new roommate, who confuses her identity with mine. When I say I'm going to take a shower and wash my hair, the woman sniffs her own underarms and asks whether she smells. She says she meant to take a shower earlier, of course she'll take one now, right away.

I force myself to put on makeup, working through gelatin, slowly, having to think of each move: *Now lift this arm*, *Now lean toward the mirror*—all habits lost, the comfort of being able to act without thought, lost.

I make three-legged stools for the kids in occupational therapy. Try to play the piano, but my fingers fail me, jerk across the keys, the keys no longer familiar. I feel like crying—is my mind, my body lost forever? But I cannot even cry.

My breasts are swollen, my abdomen swollen, my skin breaks out, I have trouble swallowing, I constantly tap my toes. What are these drugs doing to me? I feel pregnant, although I know I'm not. I ask the staff to adjust my medication—it's those pills that are making it difficult to recover.

Sam visits, arranges for us to meet on the grounds. It is mid-October, with red and gold leaves scattered on the grass, and yet it is still unseasonably warm. As I walk toward a bench, I am reminded of walking through the arboretum in my dream. He sees where I am headed and diverts us to a picnic table and sits across from me, foiling my romantic fantasies, activated now almost by habit. I hand him my written interpretations of the proverbs, and he nods, that's more like it, but I gather that still my thinking is too concrete. I want to scream in frustration.

He suggests that I return to Mount Auburn Hospital. He is more familiar with the staff there, it will be easier for Jake and the kids to visit, and that's where I started out—it might be good to return there. As if I must change the original impression I have created, return to the scene of the crime. Twice. I don't quite see why but agree anyway. Later Jake tells me Sam thinks I might be too comfortable in this scenic place, which is too much like a college dorm.

I have made many friends among the patients; I care for them, mediate between them and the staff. A woman who has seizures that may or may not be feigned; a catatonic woman released from her paralysis through shock therapy; a man, intelligent, manic-depressive, who wants to start a school, who works in education, and I inspire him with my educational theories, encourage him. The staff praise me for being such a caretaker, so helpful to others.

Before I leave, the staff and patients throw me a surprise party, an outing to see a movie and eat ice cream sundaes. We exchange phone numbers, talk about a reunion in a year. I hug so many people, say I will stay in touch. Of course I will. We are friends after all.

CHAPTER 26:

DUELING WITH THE FOG

Jake drives me to Mount Auburn. I recognize the staff, but they are now transfigured—normal, living in the present. The formerly dead roommate is anorexic, skeletally thin, and she tells me I'd scared her half to death when I'd hidden behind the door as she entered our room. A homeless woman, who insists she is the author of a major literary classic, her manuscript stolen and published under someone else's name, refers to my weaving around the ceiling lights, and says, "An intricate dance. It looked like you were doing an intricate dance."

Each morning there is a community meeting where we must identify ourselves and say why we are here. I say I didn't sleep or eat for five or six days and then became delusional, had some hallucinations. I state the facts, ignoring the why's, implying it was a mere physiological aftermath of ignoring my bodily needs. But I ask myself, Why did I stop eating, stop sleeping? Didn't the delusions come first? And if so, might it all happen again? Am I without control?

Toward the end of my stay, a male staff member tells me staff believe that if I wanted to, I could make this happen again, as if I had decided to become psychotic, that it was my choice. But it doesn't feel like that. It happened to me.

I struggle to get better and don't look at myself too closely—too ashamed of what my life has become. Instead, I focus on the other patients. I ally myself with staff as an intermediary, helping others always, walking elderly patients to staff and to the bathroom, drawing patients into conversation, doing therapy with them, becoming friends with them. It feels like home, like a womb. I have no responsibilities, the food is served, the day is structured for me. I do not want to leave. I am well-liked by all, told I am so intelligent, so insightful, so caring, they are all so sure I can have a good life, that I deserve it. Aren't I wonderful?

I have seen, in passing the staff office, my Kardex, with "depression" written on it, which I find laughable. I have been manic, euphoric, not depressed, and they know nothing of the delusions, the hallucinations, or the content of them—I have successfully kept everything to myself, with the exception of the visible manifestations—my apparently odd, inexplicable behaviors. When I ask Sam about the Kardex, he tells me they had trouble arriving at a diagnostic classification for me—they were at a loss at first, when increasingly massive doses of drugs seemed not to make a difference.

I take some computerized tests, and a woman gives me the Rorschach, the Wechsler Adult Intelligence Test, a draw-a-person test, and then asks me to take a blank piece of paper and draw my family members, each involved in a characteristic activity. Unsure what she means by "family," I decide to draw members of my family of origin, along with Jake and the kids, and am aware that the tester will look for telltale signs of pathology. When I'm happy with the drawing, I hand it to the tester and she ruins it by writing names across each character.

Later, Sam tells me she was very impressed with my drawing skill and said I could be an artist. Also that I might be manic-depressive, that maybe lithium was indicated. I say, "No, no more drugs."

Sam arrives in the early morning and wants tea. I lead him to the kitchen area, pull out a tea bag, and reach for a cup, but he edges in front of me and says he'll make his own tea, as if somehow this hospital kitchen is a bit too homey.

No one is around, so we sit at the end of the dining room table while he sips his tea. He tells me staff are concerned that I don't talk about my own issues, that I am too concerned about other patients.

I light a cigarette and look out the window. "I have to talk about you?" When he nods, yes, I do need to talk about it, I say, "So embarrassing," and shake my head slowly.

Almost all of the staff suggest I should consider changing therapists, but when I say, "You don't think he's a good therapist?" they tell me that's not the point. But when I ask Sam whether he feels he can continue to work with me, he says, "Absolutely."

He wants me to continue, I can tell, the way he visits all the time. Maybe he feels a little guilt and wants to see me through all this. And I don't want to start all over again, can't go through all this again.

I am still heavily drugged, restless, semi-paralyzed, toe-tapping, my muscles rigid. I've been given permission for my first visit home, and I sit at the kitchen table, bombarded with mechanical sounds—the buzz of the refrigerator, the creak of the chairs, the drone of the stove light.

It is lunchtime. The kids sit at the table, and Jake reads in his chair. They are waiting for me to fix lunch, I gather.

But how can I do it?

Organize the task in your mind, I order myself.

Food, what food?

I ask the kids what they want, and now I see a jumble of packages and jars with different names in my mental shopping cart, something different for each—maybe I should write it all down?

Or just get started, and they'll tell me if I make a mistake?

But how can I muster the energy to move around the kitchen, find everything, pull the food out, the dishes? Later I'll have to put it away again.

Why, oh why, doesn't Jake offer to help? Slowly I force myself to be functional, to make the lunch, the sandwiches, my anger building as he sits reading on.

After we eat, I ask Jake to take me back early. It is too much.

So drugged. My room is filled with plants, cards, gifts, among them some magazines. I flip through them but cannot read. The letters jump before my eyes, and I cannot maintain my train of thought. Am I permanently damaged? Will I ever be able to read again?

I complain about the drugs, ask to have them reduced—I would be okay if it weren't for the drugs. I ask for a meeting with the head psychiatrist, who tells me I was extremely psychotic only a few weeks ago, so the drugs are necessary, but perhaps they could try a slightly lower dose and monitor the effects.

I am again told I must discuss the issues that led to my hospitalization before I can go home, but I find that when I introduce them the other patients are irritated. They say they didn't realize I had problems. They don't want me to have needs, I think, because then how can I take care of them? They look up to me, depend on me.

I find I don't like the patients across the board, without reservation, anymore. I even cruelly mimic a couple of them to myself in their absence. I am frustrated with those who make no progress, who have not responded to the staff's help, to my help. For some reason, the closer I get to discharge, the angrier and angrier I am becoming. I wonder whether the drugs might have suppressed my emotions and made me more amiable than normal, my judgmental side now simply reemerging as those drugs are reduced.

It is the end of October. I visit home for an overnight. Opening the front door, I am struck with the mustiness, the mildew, dust, dirt. But I have longed to lie in my own bed, for the soft comfort of it in contrast to the hospital beds, which seem designed to be uncomfortable, to ensure people won't want to stay too long.

I lie in our bed, the shade slightly drawn and wonder, How can I return here? How can it ever be any different, anything other than a coffin I will die in? How can I maintain the tiny spark of hope for myself that I have developed in the hospital? That I might have something to offer to someone somewhere, to others, to the world. That I might be worthy of love, and more importantly, worthy of loving myself.

Back in the hospital, I meet with the psychiatrist again and insist I don't need medication. I know drugs are essential and helpful in many cases, but not in my individual case, at least not anymore. Now they are seriously interfering and making me dysfunctional. I am finally victorious: The doctor will have me tapered off the Haldol if I agree to take some Stelazine with me when I leave, and to use it, if necessary. I agree.

Early November. After five weeks, I am free! I walk into the house, Jake following me with my suitcase, and the kids run to me and hug me. My mother is there, shows me that she has cleaned the whole house. And then I see the roses.

"Roses! I haven't received roses since I was twenty-one." I read the card; they are from my friends.

My mother points out the carnations Jake has bought and nudges me to thank him.

I say, "Thank you. Isn't that sweet." But I think, *To my friends, I am worth roses; to Jake, yellow carnations.*

PART V:

ONWARD, 1982–

CHAPTER 27:

LEAVE-TAKINGS

Home from the hospital, I sank into depression that thinly covered a molten rage. I was still stuck in the same old life. Alone with the kids while Jake traveled, no job, no plan, no way out, and now with a stigma attached—a psychiatric history, another secret to keep.

I compulsively read murder mysteries, vicariously gratified by the murders more than the detection. I also read *If You Meet the Buddha on the Road, Kill Him!*—I was upset with Sam too, wanting him to admit some responsibility for what had happened to me. I had been shocked to discover my hospital stays would cost us about $10,000, despite Sam's earlier vague assurances that costs should be covered. On top of our store debt, it was one more burden to bear. But still I didn't directly confront him—I couldn't easily talk about my experience or the new debt, but instead focused on recovering my life, as depressing as it was.

Back in Sam's home office, I asked him, "How can I feel confident that I won't sink into psychosis again? I mean, yes, I can be sure to eat, to sleep, but this was a chicken and egg thing—why did I stop eating and sleeping in the first place? I was feeling elated, while simultaneously thinking, *I don't want to eat of this life*. But still . . ."

"You were going through a lot at the time, not taking the job, losing the store."

"No way out of an intolerable situation, yes. But also it was about Brian. And about you and me."

"It probably wasn't the best time for me to go on vacation."

"I just want to get my life back to normal. But maybe I can't. The women at the nursery school won't even let me drive in the carpool."

"How do you feel about that?"

"Patronized, but I guess I'd feel the same way if I were them. One woman asked why I'd been hospitalized, that it might help to know—maybe others had been through the same thing. I was thinking *unlikely*, but just smiled and said I'd rather not talk about it."

"You handled that well—it's your decision whether to share. And when."

He continued, "I'm interested in what else you might do to take care of yourself, in addition to eating, sleeping . . ."

I sighed. "I know it sounds grandiose, but I'd like to see if I could make some sort of career out of art or maybe writing."

"My guess is you'll probably explore any number of different career options," Sam said, as if the world was somehow wide open for me.

I was happy he believed that but had my doubts. "I know I can't do much right now, anyway, with the kids still so little. Maybe when they're both in elementary school, when childcare won't be such an expense."

I fiddled with my cigarette pack but didn't light up. "But still, can I emerge unscathed from this? Will my options be limited if people find out? I haven't talked to anyone yet about it." *Not even Sam*, I thought to myself. "It's too embarrassing—I'd look stupid and utterly ridiculous. I was crazy!"

"As a loon!" he added, and we both chuckled a little. "By the way, many people have had similar experiences and have gone on to have successful careers."

May 1983. To supplement my individual therapy with him, Sam had arranged for me to be interviewed by a group therapist, an expert in the field. When I'd been accepted into a group, back in March, Sam was excited, as if it were some kind of coup for him.

Now he leaned forward. "So how's group therapy going?"

"Still scoping it out, I guess. I haven't said much yet. But we can't afford both group and coming here, so I need to leave group."

What I didn't say was how small I felt in the group. The others were IT professionals, software designers, social workers, psychologists, a management consultant, an artist, writers, etc., and then there was me, no longer a business owner or even a volunteer nursery school treasurer. I'd been able to introduce myself at my first meeting and blurt out a little about my episode, but since then, I couldn't seem to squeeze myself into the conversations. They weren't unwelcoming, but the circle still felt closed to me—I didn't measure up.

He frowned and thought for a moment. "I'm not willing to see you individually if you won't participate in group therapy."

I was startled. Was he using my feelings for him to manipulate me?

"But I'm not really participating anyway—I can't seem to talk about my episode in there. Too embarrassing."

"I think you would benefit greatly from participating in both. You'd probably get more out of it than someone who's in psychoanalysis daily."

"I can't afford both." Why couldn't he understand that? Even if I worked part-time to pay for it, the childcare alone would eat all my earnings. I knew Jake resented paying for both, too, and I didn't feel comfortable spending money on myself, especially now that I wasn't contributing any income.

But I wasn't even making good use of my sessions with Sam—I wasn't talking about my episode with him either, except superficially, and he hadn't probed. Did it even make sense to continue with him? Was our relationship too fraught with all that was unsaid?

I decided to test the waters.

"It seems odd to me Jake has never expressed any interest in the content of my psychosis, as if he thought it was just meaningless gibberish or behavior."

"Sometimes partners don't want to know."

Still armed with my old habit, thinking Sam was cryptically referring to himself, too, I assumed he meant he didn't want to know, which rendered him just like all the other men in my life, maybe simply all the other people. It seemed a small thing—his not wanting to know—but it was what some part of me had been waiting for, the secret trigger, obliterating fantasy, moving me to flight. Not so small after all, but instead defining, the crux of it. I decided in that moment that I would leave him—that very session. If he could give me up so easily, I now had reason to do the same. Why drag out what was now clearly, incontrovertibly, inevitable?

But also I was afraid if I didn't stop seeing Sam now, I'd never get away. Since my psychotic break months before, Sam had been low-key, giving no cues that he cared about me one way or the other. He even seemed bored with me. Or maybe angry that I'd shaken his belief in himself as a successful therapist.

I sat quietly, until he asked what I was thinking.

"Since I can't afford both group and individual, today can be our last session."

His eyes widened, and he winced, as if in pain. "Most people take eight or ten months to terminate."

At his request, I did drag it out for two more weeks. He wanted Jake to come to our next session, for closure. My last individual session was coincidentally on Brian's birthday. And on that day eight years before, I'd left graduate school. I thought of mentioning it, but we weren't there to talk about Brian anymore.

Sam asked, "If you had sufficient income in the future, do you think you might return to individual therapy?"

He'd asked something like that the previous week. Why was he asking again? Hardening my heart, I said, "No, there are other things we need to spend money on."

"I must admit this is a hard session for me. Most people take much longer to terminate."

I tried to lighten the moment by laughing and saying I was just impulsive by nature, but when he grimaced, I saw I'd failed.

When he stood and it was time to say goodbye, I wondered if I could finally hug him, but he stood at a distance I couldn't quite cross, so I extended my hand. He shook it, squeezing it twice, just as in the hospital, and commented that I had a lot going for me.

And then to my surprise, he walked me down the stairs and to the door, as if he meant he was willing to leave the room with me, my old fantasy.

I turned to him and said, "In case I don't see you again, I hope you have a good life."

He said, "I'll give it a good shot."

This time *I* winced. All I could think of was Brian, giving himself a good shot. Why would Sam say such a thing to me? And then I was driving my Bug to the end of the dead-end street, and when I turned around, I saw him still standing in the doorway watching me, and I gunned my engine and zoomed away, as if I were making a grand escape.

It was only after leaving Sam that I allowed myself to feel the significance of what I'd done. At odd moments I felt the weight of my hasty decision and teared up, feeling I'd made a terrible mistake. I wrote letters to him—in my journal. Unsent.

A week or two after leaving him, while I was driving to group, I saw a green Saab with bumper stickers not far ahead of me—Sam's car, driving a little erratically. Just as I was about to turn left to the leader's house, I saw him adjusting his rearview mirror and then looking quickly in his side mirror. Was it a coincidence? Or a plan? He knew when and where the meetings were held. If a coincidence, did he now think I was following him? I was sad to think this ambiguous moment might be the last time I'd ever see him.

In a group session, I talked about leaving Sam, how I couldn't afford both group and individual therapy, and they mostly agreed with Sam, that I could have found a way to do both, which meant they too didn't understand exactly how little money we had. I already felt guilty about spending so much for my cigarettes.

Or, of course, they knew it was *not* just about money, but I had trouble talking about it. I was hurt that, if Sam did have feelings for me, he hadn't chosen to be with me, hadn't chosen me, even though I understood that if he had, the cost might have been too great for him, the ethical compromise, the self-inflicted stain on his own self-image. And a burden no relationship would likely survive. In the end, I didn't want to hurt him or me and knew on some level I had to leave. But my heart was slower to let him go. I thought of him often, dreamt about him.

I began to look forward to group therapy each week. Once I became more familiar with other members, it felt safer to talk. The leader didn't prohibit socializing among group members, and a number of us would go to dinner after our sessions (where I'd order only an appetizer to save money), and some ended up becoming close friends, my chosen family. Group therapy was a great setting for challenging my beliefs about myself and to learn how others saw me, while also learning about how others dealt with their own issues and helping each other along the way. And I liked the reciprocity.

Most sessions were helpful, but one in particular highlighted my own driven nature. A man about my age, early thirties, used the phrase "the pressure I feel as a man to achieve something with my life" and I flew into a rage and interrupted him, "You think that's only the province of men?! I've always felt immense internal pressure to accomplish something significant with my life, something meaningful." That was my mission, I thought to myself.

I was pleased when other people chimed in, both women and men, to support my position.

During the next three years, I did, as Sam predicted, explore different career options. I started drawing detailed portraits with charcoal pencil, first of family members and some actors (to show I could capture likenesses), and after some marketing effort, I drew portraits by commission. After about a year, I had enough drawings for a solo show at the Watertown Library.

When I realized my artistic efforts were unlikely to create an income that would allow me to leave Jake, I again considered returning to school and becoming a therapist, but I thought it would help to have some clinical experience first to beef up my application. I talked the head of a Brookline psychiatric hospital into hiring me as a mental health worker even though she thought I was overqualified. Because the hours were 7:00 a.m. to 3:00 p.m., I needed minimal childcare, and our landlady, who lived above us, agreed to do it.

I did worry about running into doctors/staff who might know me from those five weeks when I was a patient only two years earlier, and then it happened—one of the emergency room doctors from Belmont Hospital appeared in the unit. But if he did recognize me, he said nothing. My therapy group members assured me there were plenty of practicing psychotherapists who had been through experiences like mine without losing their careers.

I worked at the hospital for nine months, talking with patients and leading a creative writing group, but left the job because I didn't feel I was making a meaningful impact, and so I also ruled out a career as a therapist.

Before my psychotic episode, I'd been planning to write about my peak experience, how the world was permeated with meaning, how my perceptions changed. I'd been writing in a journal for years, had written short stories, and had exchanged some with a couple of the writers in my therapy group. Now I wondered whether I could write a book about the peak experience and my episode. Group members encouraged me, and some said it sounded like an intriguing read.

When an old friend from grad school, now a therapist, visited Massachusetts and met me for coffee, I told her about my episode, despite my feelings of shame. She reacted by saying she wished she could have an experience like mine, to know what it was like from the inside—that it could be helpful in working with her clients.

I'd been feeling it was humiliating to have become psychotic even if it was transitory, that it was something I would always be embarrassed to share, and it was, but now her comment led me to reframe it—because it was, in fact, a fascinating experience, and writing about it could be valuable to others. Its value wouldn't lie in describing my particular life per se, but in showing how it could happen, what it was like from the inside, and how ultimately it could be life-changing.

Ignoring what would likely be Jake's reaction, I bought an electronic typewriter. Jake surprised me by not becoming angry—he believed I could write the book. For a few months, I wrote about my peak experience and psychotic episode, using notes from my journals. I tried not to think about whether it would ever be publishable or whether I would dare to have it published. I just had to get it on paper.

1986. Jake and I were leading those parallel lives we had depicted in sculptures for Sam four years earlier. Still married, still living in the same apartment, but seeing each other in passing. While I understood this period as a pause, until the kids were older and we could afford to split up, Jake thought otherwise.

It was Valentine's Day. Jake had come home with a Valentine's card for me that said, "I still love you, and I don't want it to be this way." I was enraged—he was refusing to accept it was over, despite repeated arguments. I tore through some desk drawers, found a deserted green envelope, licked it shut, and took it to him.

"Here's your Valentine from me," I said, and stuck it in his face.

A little smile curved his lips, and his eyes softened. He said, "For me?"

And as he was ripping it open, I gritted my teeth and said, "This is what I have for you—nothing. Nothing at all!"

"You're being too—" Jake said, with a grimace.

"No! Don't say it." Why did he force me to be so mean? To be just like my mother. Why couldn't he accept that it was over?

As we continued to argue, I heard whimpering from near the kitchen sink, and then wailing, and I stopped and looked around the counter and saw Brandon, covering his five-year-old ears with pudgy hands, terrified, and crying, "No, no, no." Jessie, almost eight, sat on the piano bench in the next room, swinging her legs hard, pretending to read a book. How could I ever forgive myself for traumatizing the kids like that?

Still, I believed the kids would be better off in a happy home, even if it meant some initial pain for all of us. I decided it was ludicrous to hope so fervently that I could generate enough income with my art or writing to allow me to leave Jake. And I couldn't wait until I had a job—too easy to defer finding one. I would simply leap into the unknown, force myself into a position where I would have to make changes to survive. I'd already waited three years for both kids to be in school.

I filed for divorce, and together Jake and I told the children. As they cried, I steeled myself away, my feelings residing in a hard lump situated just below my breastbone. I waited until it was over, endured in that small place inside of me until Jake was gone.

I thought he would leave that day, walk out, but he didn't. He stayed for months, refusing to believe it was over. It was only when I said I would then leave both him and the children that he finally left in a jiffy.

Jake was the only man in the courtroom. I wondered how he felt, surrounded by so much estrogen. The judge refused to sign the agreement until more child support was added, but even then said she thought it was a poor deal for me (and probably also that I was a fool)—with no job and no immediate prospects. And I was a fool, but at least I was free, free at last.

CHAPTER 28:

JOINING THE DANCE

After five long months of struggling to find a job, while relying on my first credit card to meet living expenses, my unusual combination of skills—my experience as a grad school teaching assistant, mental health counselor, business owner, bookkeeper accountant/nursery school treasurer, and writer—led to my hire as director of a skills training program for displaced homemakers and single mothers much like myself. I administered the program, wrote proposals, budgeted, hired and supervised staff, taught career development, developed internships in high-tech firms, counseled trainees, and helped place them in jobs. Years later, I occasionally ran into former trainees who said I'd changed their lives. I was happy to see how well they were doing and thrilled to hear I'd helped them along the path to more satisfying lives.

Being a single parent, while working full-time and managing all the usual household tasks, was a constant struggle. Cobbling together after-school, vacation, and summer childcare and figuring out how to handle the kids' school activities, illnesses, and accidents (a pencil impaled in the sole of Brandon's foot, Jessie's allergic reaction to a bee sting, and the worst, when

Jessie was struck by a car) was a source of persistent stress. But at least I had a professional life that allowed me to feel competent and productive.

When the kids were in their early teens, I joined an evening writing group and worked on an entire rewrite of my book for a couple of years, but couldn't yet contemplate publication—I was too worried about the impact the revelation of past mental illness might have on my reputation and career. Very few people knew about my experience. Other than my closest friends when I was hospitalized and members of my therapy and writing groups, I'd told no one.

For me, 1995 was a banner year. After fourteen years of trying to give up smoking, I'd been scared into quitting. The kids and I were living in a three-bedroom townhouse, and one afternoon, while I was home alone, I was looking in the mirror of our downstairs bathroom when suddenly I was unable to breathe—my lungs simply did not work. I lurched out of the bathroom, terrified, pounding at my chest, and tried to give myself the Heimlich maneuver by throwing myself against the kitchen sink, although there was nothing in my throat. Finally, I gasped and inhaled with relief.

I'd felt utterly helpless, as though some force had assumed control of my body, and I attributed it to smoking. After that shock, quitting seemed clearly a matter of life and death. I chewed Nicorette, tapering down until I was finally free.

I ultimately became executive director of a regional workforce board, comprised of business leaders, educators, training providers, and state and community representatives working together to oversee the use of funds to help unemployed men and women access training and develop careers. It was meaningful work, providing support to people at those critical junctures when they were feeling most vulnerable and possibly as lost as Brian and I had once felt.

Moonlighting as a consultant, I also designed performance reports for the state career center system that I'd helped establish. For fun, I helped people from around the world solve problems in designing Crystal Reports through a popular online forum where users thanked me with thousands of little purple stars, commenting at times that I'd saved their jobs or even their lives.

After thirty years in the workforce development field, I retired on Brian's birthday, 2016. Six months earlier, I'd been browsing realty in Western Massachusetts to see what kind of condo I could afford if I left the Boston area when I retired, though I didn't know then when that might be. I stumbled upon a four-level townhouse in a former paper mill and fell in love with it. The BAILEY'S IRISH CREAM sign (sporting my name) in the loft bar seemed an omen—the condo was meant to be mine, although the bar would have to go—I hadn't had a drink since that Thanksgiving, 1981.

Just weeks later, I bought the townhouse, gave six months' notice to the board, and started prepping my three-bedroom house for sale. While I wanted to live closer to my kids, I hadn't specifically planned to move to the exact town where they both lived—that the condo I loved was located there was serendipitous.

It was April 2023. Jessie and Brandon were coming over for taco night in a few hours. I looked out my ten-foot windows onto a hill garden lush with flowers and shrubs, a dogwood and an old spruce, and marveled at how grateful I felt for the life I had now. I had just shipped an oil portrait to my childhood best friend, a painting of her granddaughters in fairy costumes. Earlier, I'd painted a portrait of Brian at twenty-one, using a rare photo of him as an adult, but plugging in his Austin-Healey and an ocean view—what might be a happy place. I thought seeing him on my wall might be upsetting, but instead, I felt I'd brought him alive in some way.

Another painting, "Family Reunion," showed Mandy and me sorting through the apple box of Brian's things, while the ghosts of Brian (sitting on the hearth, holding a rifle), our now deceased mother (draped in a white gown, with wild black hair surrounding her white streak, and suspended from a brick wall), and late father (reading a book on the sofa) look on.

Hank, my longtime love, had commissioned several paintings, as had some of his friends/family and others. He lived a couple hours away, but was coming for the weekend in a few days. Not living together had, maybe not so surprisingly, kept the romance alive. I enjoyed my time alone and not having to adapt to a partner's needs on a regular basis.

While waiting for the kids to arrive, I sat down and opened my Mac to resume another edit of my book. Mandy, who would be visiting from Montana next month, had been my first reader, and I wanted her to take another look after this revision.

It was the story of Brian and me, our lives intertwined, then diverging; of two lives gone astray, one ended, one restored. When I'd felt trapped in an intolerable situation, desperate for a life for myself, but equally unable to abandon my kids, I was squeezed into the only way out—my own alternative reality. My craziness extracted me from my untenable life situation, just like those claws in the arcade that capture the prize stuffed animal. It was in fact a safety valve, and might have been for Brian too. He had, after all, committed suicide only when he seemed on the mend, when he had the capacity to think clearly, due to medication, and consider his own future—one that looked impossible to him because he believed his mind was permanently altered, that he'd never be himself again. As wrongheaded as that might have been.

Similarly, my five-week hospitalization was another extraction—it took me out of my environment and exposed me to people who surprised me by seeing me differently than I saw myself, who reminded me of my own capabilities, who even admired me.

My book was also the story of Sam and me, and how our therapeutic relationship had contributed to my episode. While I found his enigmatic comments intriguing, they also led me to wonder constantly what he *really* meant and, in turn, what he felt about me. I felt safe with him more than with anyone, but at the same time, because I couldn't know everything about him, I felt vulnerable, afraid I might learn that he didn't even like me. My obsessive need to know how he felt about me was partly a defense mechanism, maybe to drive him away, but also part of me wanted to know if I could be fully known and still loved.

I hear the transference bells ringing, and I say *absolutely*. A straight line could be drawn between my persistent attempts to earn my mother's love and my feelings for Sam. But does that mean I didn't "really" love him?

What is transference? If defined as a displacement of feelings onto the therapist that originated in relation to other significant figures in one's life, does it mean those feelings are less real if generated in the therapeutic setting? Or somehow maladaptive? After all, who we are as individuals and how we love others is absolutely shaped by those significant others. How else do we learn how to feel, to react to others?

I would argue that I did know who Sam was as a person, by the way he related to me (and sometimes Jake) in the room. I didn't know all the facts, the ins and outs, of his life, e.g., how he behaved in a social setting, but I could make a good guess, and I did know more than most clients do through Jake's previous association with him. That in itself blurred the boundaries.

That Sam felt he couldn't tell me his feelings added to my distress—I felt so close to having the love I wanted. Of course, I always found ways to creatively interpret what he said to discourage me so I could maintain hope. Even in my "craziness," some part of me knew living out my dream of running away with Sam probably wouldn't end well—the sun and the moon may never meet. But I do think the ambiguity in our relationship was a key factor in my breakdown.

A year after leaving therapy, I called him one last time and invited him to see my show at the library. Then I asked, "Do you think we could have coffee sometime, just to talk?"

He hesitated, then quietly said, "I'd have to think about that."

"I'm still having trouble letting go. I know it's foolish."

"We had a very powerful relationship."

"I guess I want you to say no so I can give up these fantasies I still have of you and me. I want you to tell me you were never in love with me. Please just say those words."

Quietly he said, "I was never in love with you."

I teared up, but thanked him and said goodbye.

He'd said we'd had a very powerful relationship, and that validated what I'd felt. I finally felt a sense of closure, even though I'd orchestrated his words. I'd loved him and was grateful for my time with him. I came to understand our relationship as a necessary entanglement, encapsulating for me the kind of deep connection I'd longed for. He had sustained me at my lowest point, bolstered that little white light, fanned it back into a flame.

Looking over the arc of my life, it's easy to see that I looked to men when I couldn't bear to face my own lost self. First Ian, then Jake, and Sam, when what I needed was to find, accept, and value myself. In some ways, Ian and Jake both were collateral damage as I struggled to identify and carve out the life I wanted, the life I needed. They were good guys in many ways—I loved each of them at one time and still think of them fondly.

My peak/psychotic experience and hospitalization, in fact, jump-started my own belief in myself and my exploration of the life I might be able to have. So in a way it was a gift. Yet, I still found it difficult to talk about my experience—it was one thing to write about it in a book, with readers at some distance, and another to tell my neighbors and friends that my book was about my own psychotic episode and about falling in love with my therapist in particular—it was so cliché and felt like a personal failing. I didn't even tell those closest to me until recent years. I was relieved to discover they still appeared to care about me and didn't immediately start looking for pathology, that I still had value in their eyes.

I wanted them to continue to see a woman of strength and substance, not an empty vessel to be filled by others' perceptions or expectations of me. A complex woman who was now ready to share her story, in the hope that it might give someone else the motivation to persist through tough times.

Of course, *every* individual is complex, a thousand- or million-piece puzzle with multicolored, variously shaped pieces that tell a unique story. I'm reminded of my dream when I was first home from the hospital, over forty years ago:

> *I'm in the psychology department at Berkeley. In my mailbox, I find an envelope containing a picture of six dancers, with the fourth one from the left missing, an empty outline of the dancer shown instead. I'm being invited by Dr. Manfred, my grad school advisor, to become the fourth dancer. I walk down the hall and find a stage on the left with the dancers, and to the right, a giant (12' by 12') puzzle of a city—not a map, but a picture. Dr. Manfred, who stands next to me, tells me I am supposed to put it together—although it is already assembled.*

I understood that I myself was the city, in all its aspects, the heights of the skyscrapers, the dark alleys, the twisted streets, the bustling activity, the noise, the music, the niches of anger, solitude, joy and sorrow, good and bad—already assembled inside me.

And what was the dance I was invited to join? Perhaps immersion in some act that could unite being and doing to create something beyond self. For me, it was my writing, painting, and sometimes plain old problem-solving. My desperate search for Sam, for my rightful home, was a search not just for a deep, mutual love, a reciprocal experience of feeling fully known and still loved, but for a life that could engage and sustain me.

Finally, I was home. I had called my own number, answered, and accepted my own invitation.

My reverie was broken by the sound of knocking. Jessie and Brandon had arrived.

ACKNOWLEDGMENTS

My unending and heartfelt thanks to:

My terrific editors, also published authors themselves, who each in their own way helped me find the story and write a better book: Jodi Fodor, Michele Orwin, DM Gordon, and Dori Ostermiller.

Brooke Warner and Crystal Patriarche and their respective teams for their expertise and guidance along the way.

Jenna Russo, an invaluable and insightful critic, cheerleader, and incidental comedian.

Marcia Booth, Darlene Basmajian, and Judy Kane, early readers who were generous with their praise, while also helping clarify what was and wasn't working, and who helped me believe the story was worthy of being told.

Jane Barnes and Ann Wadsworth, who read an earlier version in our long-ago "Fayerweather Friends" writing group.

George Moriarty, for lending his ear and unwavering support and for his uplifting sense of humor.

Sue Tippett, for her insight, clarity, and steadfast encouragement.

Finally, my friends and family, those I've loved both then and now.

ABOUT THE AUTHOR

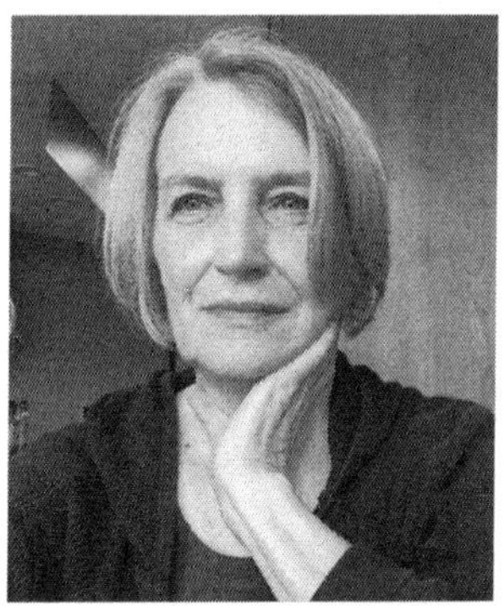

Linda Bass grew up in Wisconsin before moving to California, where she earned a BA in psychology from UCLA and an MA in psychology from UC Berkeley. She worked in the workforce development field for thirty years, most recently as the executive director of a regional workforce board in Cambridge, Massachusetts, and also worked as a Crystal Reports designer on a consulting basis. After retiring, she moved to Western Massachusetts, where she spends her time writing and painting, solving puzzles, reading, singing (to herself), enjoying friends and family, and feeling grateful for all of it. She is currently working on a second book.

Her author website: lindabass.com

Her art website: lindabassart.com